Vital Health Bio Assessment Guide

CUTTING EDGE ASSESSMENT TECHNOLOGY FOR HEALTH PROFESSIONALS

David S. Lee

VITAL HEALTH BIO ASSESSMENT GUIDE:
CUTTINGEDGEASSESSMENTTECHNOLOGY
FOR HEALTH PROFESSIONALS
by David S. Lee.

ISBN 9780994922236

In memory
of my dear mentor and
friend Julian Beecroft

Table of Contents

www.vitalhealthlife.com

Acknowledgements

I would like to deeply thank the following people:
Irfaan Haniff for doing a fabulous job in editing the definition section of the Bio-results section of the book.

Rohit Bhatia for being such a reliable business partner in getting some of the work done to finish this book.

Dusan Misic for excellent work in the formatting and design of the book layout.

My teachers at the International Academy of Natural Health Science, especially John Freeman, Cecile Savereux and Dr. Dorothy Marshall, for their encouraging and insightful teachings; Dr. George Grant for guiding me through his vast knowledge of medical science and nutritional biochemistry;

Todd Norton for his friendship, encouragement and input on health issues and bio-nutritional facts; Tonie and Luis Rivas for being there as friends and supporting me in various health endeavours;

Bill Garbarino for his friendship, steadfast guidance, and wise business counsel over the years through the various circumstances and development of Vital Health;

My dear sister, Ella, who always believed in me, supported my vision and encouraged me during those challenging times in my life when I had to clarify my dreams;

My late mentor and friend, James Stockton, who was like an earthly Christ figure in my life, who impacted my thoughts and life with not just his wise words but his everyday example of loving people and giving;

And my late mentor and father figure, Julian, who exposed me to whole foods and thought provoking ideas; and for birthing many of the health and fitness ideas which I later developed further into the Vital Health System.

Preface

I wrote this book to help Health Professionals have an additional tool and system of giving their clients a more detailed health assessment, so their work in coming up with the right program, solution or procedure would be that much more effective in helping to enhance the health state of their clients.

Introduction

There are about 30 trillion cells in the adult body. Most of them divide and renew themselves. At the atomic level of each cell, the nucleus and the electrons are changing at high speeds. As they do this, they radiate electromagnetic waves constantly outward. Each cell of the body, whether it be in a healthy, sub-healthy or diseased state has a different corresponding electromagnetic wave. Hence, if the group of cells of a particular organ or system of the body has a different electromagnetic wave, then this will be picked up by the Quantum Resonance device, and interpreted through its program and given the appropriate readings. The frequency and the energy of the magnetic field is measured by the Quantum Resonance device through the sensor of the hand-held probe.

This book not only goes into and covers the Interpretation of the Quantum Resonance results of the client's various body's systems, but it also will explain and cover the three other health assessments that have been developed by the author so that when you as a health practitioner does an assessment of your client's health, you get to see a broader view of the lifestyle related to the results, the person's health history, activities, state of mind, etc.. Hence you can get a better picture of your client's health state, so you can give a more accurate recommendation towards coming up with a solution for them.

INSTALLATION INSTRUCTIONS

Insert the CD/DVD ROM into the drive reader and the installation process will start automatically. (If not, go into the disc file, and double click the document Setup.exe file) The program will run on Windows as the following Welcome page displays on your screen. Click "Next" to go to the next step. The different installation pages will appear. Keep clicking "Next" until it displays the "Finish" button. As mentioned in the device manual, the program will install and work on Windows 98/Me System with the Microsoft Office program on it for it to run normally. If it is installed in 2000/XP/Vista System it will work without any other software support. After the install program has finished, the icon of the Quantum Resonance Magnetic Analyzer should appear on your desktop. If not, check in your main drive folders for the program icon and make a desktop shortcut for it.

In order to run the program and install it you need to insert the USB stick that came with your device which has corresponding programs on it to help run the program. Also make sure you attach the USB cable from your PC or laptop to the device input. In addition connect the probe handle into the device as well before you start the program to test your client.

OPERATION OF THE PROGRAM

Once the program icon is on your desktop click on it until it is open. Then click on "Dossier" in the toolbar which gives you the tested record of client information or profile. Tested records means scanned reports of clients from past. On the left bar of page the client and group list is displayed. Here the client and group records can be managed, edited, deleted and searched for. You can click the "Add" button under the Client records to add new client in-formation so they can be tested with the scan.

The Group Records function can divide customers into several groups. You can click "Add" to create new group, "Save" to store new group and click "Edit" to modify the name of the group. You can also click "Delete" to erase the group. If there are any members in the group, they must be first deleted, and then the group can be deleted.

After the new client has been added to the client list, connect the device to the computer if you already have done so and click on "Testing" on the toolbar and the testing page will appear. Click the "Start" button and the page will indicate to hold the rod by left hand for males and right hand for females. You click "Start Test" and the testing process will begin. It takes about 56 seconds and a pop up will indicate that "Testing is Complete". A "Testing Record Management" page should appear. Click "Get Report" which will process and open the report of the results from the test of the client. It's important to save this report onto your hard drive for future records of your client. This way, you can even email results to your client if you wish. Most clients want the result emailed to them. This greatly adds value to the service of the assessment. Also, you can "Delete" the report at this stage or compare reports tested at different times. You have to always "Get Report" before using the "Comparative" function. Click on "Full Page" function for a full page view, "Print" to print the report, "Save Report" to save the report onto your computer as a zip file. "Return" will take you back to the "Tested Record Interface".

Furthermore, you can click the "Compositive Report" which shows a summary report of all the results of the various components of the client's body that has abnormal readings. On the right of this report, a list of suggestions is given. You may notice many of the recommendations are different from the western diet. The reason for this is that the devices are manufactured in China so their cultural foods and recommendations are mentioned. You can edit and add to this suggestion section according to your nutritional methods. Use this as part of your nutritional resource for your client.

SYSTEM SETTING

This function is used for setting some of the features of the report satisfying the client's requirements. The three settings are:

Display Report Setting:
- Client can choose the report according to their requirement, and block some unnecessary report.

Preferences:
- You can choose different parameters of the report. The parameters can be shown or hidden according to customer's need.

Sensitivity Adjustment:
- You can adjust the sensitivity of the detecting rod. If you have a hard time detecting some health issues for a client's report, you can increase the sensitivity. However, it is usually best to leave it at maximum sensitivity.

BIO-ASSESSMENT PROCEDURE

1. Before you assess the client, check the computer, the device, the printer and make sure all cables are connected. Check the detecting rod is inserted tightly. Also make certain all USB and CD/DVD drives are operating or the program will not work properly.
2. Enter the client's basic information (e.g. name, gender, birthday and so on)
3. Ask client to stay relaxed and to concentrate on their breathing. Do not talk while holding the detection rod and while the device is assessing for the minute. Your voice frequency may disrupt the frequency reading of the device.
4. The detecting room should be quiet, clean and tidy.
5. Ask the client to remove excessive jewellery, phones, beepers and any communication devices off their body.
6. People with a pacemaker cannot be assessed.
7. The client is asked to gently hold the detecting rod with either left or right hand.
8. During the detecting process, the detected person's skin should not be touched.
9. Clean the rod after use so people's skin oils and sweat is wiped off the detecting rod.
10. After use, make sure you put away the Quantum device in a good, secure place where it will not get damaged or get dirty.

PRECAUTIONS FOR CLIENTS

- Do not ingest alcohol, coffee or any health supplements on the day of the Bio-assessment. Furthermore, do not eat any food or take any medicine at least four hours before the Bio-scan. Also it's best for women who are on any kind of birth control pill to come in for the scan on the days they are not taking the pill. Since this may affect the hormone levels in the body which will change the hormone readings of the Bio-scan.
- Have a good night's sleep.
- If you have done some sort of intense sport activity, take a one- to two-hour rest before the scanning appointment.
- Clothes should be loose and warm enough to keep your body temperature stable.
- Do not talk while being scanned for the minute.

MAINTENANCE

- The software/hardware of the device should be installed according to the instructions of the device manual.
- The analyzer device is sensitive, so avoid any collision of any kind.
- Do not put the device in a high temperature, humid, corrosive or radioactive place. Avoid direct sunlight.
- The detecting rod should be cleaned after use with a soft cloth or cotton ball.
- The wire of the detecting rod should not be over stretched in any way as to avoid damage.

Vital Health Assessments

HEALTH CONSULT SHEET

This is a health intake sheet where you get a basic picture of your client's healthy history and current state of health. It begins with their contact information and age, weight and height. This allows you to see if they are overweight for their height. Also, taking note of age will allow you to give better guidance, since at certain ages we are more susceptible to certain conditions as a female or as a male. You will also want to know about their physical activities. This gives you an indication of whether they are motivated about exercising and allows you to gage their fitness level. If they downhill ski regularly and mountain bike, for example, they may lose weight more easily with a better meal plan. They may also be able to feel the difference in their strength and endurance, based on foods consumed before activity.

The client will then fill out the section on "What health and fitness benefits they most like to accomplish". This section will allow you to see what they want to focus on if they follow up with a program with you on nutrition and/or health services. If they check off many of the benefits in the list, it may indicate they are open and ready to sign on to your program and services.

The section covering health issues is important. This allows you to see what kind of conditions your client is dealing with, if any. This will help you determine which nutritional plan or health service package will be the best fit for them, so they get the best results.

The next section is the Goal list, where they need to indicate what their top two or three health goals are, such as "losing weight", "increase energy", "decrease acid indigestion", etc... They also need to give each goal a rating so you can see how important each goal is. This is good information to have when you present your health services and the associated costs. If the client has second thoughts, you can remind them of the high rating they wrote for their health goal. This may help them to stay focused on the importance of their health and why they came to you.

The last section of the health consult sheet covers the personal aspects of the client, such as "Why" do they want to achieve their goal. The more you can help them clarify and explain their "Why", the more they will likely stick to your health program. Included will be information about what kind of support they have in regards to sticking to a healthy lifestyle, healthy eating habits, etc. Also, it's good to know what they are looking for from you in particular. Do they want you to be direct and keep them accountable in their eating, taking that green smoothie recipe or doing their postural exercises for their spine, etc.?

NUTRITION FOOD SCORE

The next assessment is the food score sheet where the client fills out a sheet on what they eat and drink for a given day from morning till bedtime. They should also indicate how much water they drink throughout the day and give the approximate portion size of food in ounces. If they eat quite differently on the weekends compared to during the week, then you should have them fill out two Food Score sheets; one for weekday meals and another for the weekend.

FLUIDS

Once it's filled out, you can assess the basic aspects of the nutrition.

The first is how much water are they drinking per day? To get the recommended amount you divide their bodyweight by 2 and that should give you the amount they need in ounces for their bodyweight. For example, if they weigh 160 pounds, divide 160 by 2 which gives you 80 ounces. Then you would divide by 8 which would give you the number of cups of water they should have per day. In addition, look at the rating score legend at the top of the score sheet that gives the different number ratings for each component of the nutrition content of the foods your client is consuming. In this case, if the client was drinking 10 cups of water per day, then you give them an average score of 3 in the box column to show they are getting the average amount of water they need. However, if they are drinking 12 cups, then you would give them a score of 4 for above average. If they are only drinking 6 cups per day, then they should receive a score of 2. If they drink only 4 cups a day, then the score would be 1.

VITAMINS & MINERALS

If they are taking a one-a-day multi-vitamin and mineral tablet, I would give them a score of 1. If they are taking a B-complex capsule, tsp of Vitamin C powder, 350 mg capsule of Calcium & Magnesium and two soft gel capsules of Omega-3 oil in the morning with their breakfast, I would give them a score of 3, for average. If, in addition to all the mentioned supplements, they also take a heaping tsp of a concentrated green powder like Greens Plus, a half tsp of pure Chlorella powder, and 2 scoops of a quality vegetarian or whey isolate powder protein shake, I would give them a score of 4, for above average.

DEPLETING PROTEINS

If they consume mainly processed meats like bacon, side bacon, non-free-range eggs, nitrate-preserved deli meats, farmed fish, non-organic chicken and beef, I would give them a score of 3 to 4, for average or above average intake for Depleting Proteins. If they consume at least one meal a day of organic meat, wild fish or free-range eggs along with the rest of the protein for the day as mentioned, I would give them a score of 2, for Depleting Proteins.

BUILDING PROTEINS

For Building Proteins, they should consume mainly organic meats, free-range eggs, nitrate free, preservative-free deli meats, wild fish, organically fed, free-range chicken and beef for a score of 3 to 4. If they consume at least one meal a day of organic meat, wild fish or free-range eggs along with the rest of the protein for the day as mentioned, I would give them a score of 2 to 3, depending on how much processed protein sources they ate per meal verses organic protein sources.

ENZYME LEVEL

For Enzyme Level, determine how many times throughout the day your client is eating some portion of raw vegetables such as carrots, celery, cucumbers, lettuce, bell peppers, as well as raw fruit. These contain enzymes which help digest food and nourish the body along with hundreds of phytochemicals. If the client consumes around 2 to 3 servings of fruit a day and 2 to 3 servings of raw vegetables, in the form of a salad or on its own, I give them a score of 3, for average. If they consume only 1 serving of fruit and 1 serving of raw vegetables, I give them a score of 2 or less depending how large the portion. If a person is consuming more than 2 to 3 servings of vegetables and fruits and a natural multi-enzyme supplement, I would give them a score of 4, for above average.

UNHEALTHY CARBOHYDRATES

If a client is eating 2 to 3 servings of carbohydrates such as inorganic multi-grain bread, but that still has white flour mixed into it, and are eating baked goods every few days made from white flour and refined sugar, their unhealthy carbohydrates score is a 3, for average. If they are consuming 3 or more servings of unhealthy carbohydrates for the day, the score should be a 4. If they are just having a slice or two of the multi-grain bread for breakfast, the score would be around 1 or 2 for unhealthy carbohydrates.

HEALTHY CARBOHYDRATES

When a client is consuming 1 slice of organic bread, one serving sweet potatoes and one serving of brown rice for the day, the score would be a 3 for average. If the client eats more than these portions for each carbohydrate mentioned then they would get a score of 4. If client consumes less than the average portion of healthy crabs mentioned then they would receive a score of 2 or less depending on the portion size and frequency. Other forms of healthy crabs are whole wheat pasta, rice noodles, brown rice, millet, quinoa, and organic oats.

FIBER

The recommended amount of fiber for adults is around 25 to 30 grams per day. If the client consumes one medium potato and 8 ounces of brown rice for the day, they should receive a score of 3. If they eat more than these amounts, I give them a score of 4 and if they eat less than these amounts, I usually give the client a score of 2 or less. Here is a short list of foods high in fiber1:

2 oz brown rice	7 g
1 medium potato	5 g
4 oz almonds	8 g
1 medium apple	4 g
1 avocado	12 g
1 whole wheat pita	5 g
4 oz Brazil nuts	4 g
4 oz steamed carrots	3 g
8 oz natural grain cereal 7 g	

HEALTHY FATS

If the client consumes at least 3 servings of healthy fat foods per day, I give them a score of 3, for average. If they consume more than this, I give a score of 4, for above average, and if they consume less than this, I give them a score of 2 or less. Some of the healthy fat foods are avocado, cheese, whole eggs, nuts, chia seeds, olive oil, and fatty fish like salmon.

UNHEALTHY FATS

When a client consumes foods high in saturated fat 2 times per day, I give them a score of 4, for above average. If they eat only one serving of foods made with unhealthy fats per day, I give them a score of 3, for average. Some of the unhealthy fat foods are bacon, pork sausage, fried beef, deep fried foods, french fries, processed cheese and salad dressings using pasteurized canola oil.

HORMONAL HEALTH PROFILE

Glands and tissues manufacture, deliver and process various hormones that take on the role of chemical messengers that activate communication processes throughout the body. Your thoughts, feelings, the meal you ate last night, the depth of your breathing, your exercise activity, amount of coffee you drank, your attraction to a person and your enjoyment of sex all have an impact on your hormones. Hormones affect how you look, how much fat verses muscle composition you have, feel of your skin texture, and hair health. They also help stimulate your metabolism, ability to lose fat, feel calmer, sleep better, get stronger, feel sexier and focus better. Since hormones control our appetite and metabolism, maintaining hormonal balance has an important role in effective fat loss. Diet and exercise play a role, but so does sleeping well, reducing toxin exposure, healthy liver function, optimal digestion, limiting stress and decreasing inflammation. All of this influences our body in keeping our hormones in balance and losing weight.2

This Hormonal Health Profile sheet will allow you to gather information as to where your client is in terms of whether their hormone level is too high or too low. This will allow you to figure out which foods, lifestyle habits and supplements to introduce to bring the hormone level to a healthy balance.

INFLAMMATION

The inflammation level in the body also helps us to determine what is going on. This section of the profile will tell you if your client is experiencing a high degree of inflammation. A certain level is normal, as in a sinus infection from a cold, swelling from a sprained knee or a skin rash response to an allergy. However, consistent inflammation can lead to tissue destruction and disease. This is the root of diseases associated with aging. Illnesses like

arthritis, cancer, heart disease, obesity; osteoporosis, Alzheimer's, autoimmune disease, diabetes and stroke have all been initiated from inflammation in the body.3

Some of the main causes of inflammation are centered on digestion and 60 percent of the immune system is based on your digestive health. Therefore, food allergies, bacterial imbalance, deficiency of enzymes or acids, yeast overgrowth, parasites and stress affect our digestion and cause inflammation which affects our immune system. In addition, gas, bloating, heartburn, acid reflux, constipation, diarrhea, IBS, Crohn's and ulcerative colitis are the common digestive conditions. These can be greatly turned around by increasing the good bacterial count, identifying the allergic foods, identifying missing enzymes and increasing them, following food-combining principles that decrease acidity, as well as introducing more alkaline foods, such as green vegetables like kale, spinach, and Swiss chard. Cutting out breads, sugars and acidic foods to decrease yeast in the body is recommended, as well as deep parasite cleanses using quality natural herbal supplements and making changes in lifestyle to decrease stress levels. Furthermore, exercising regularly produces anti-inflammatory compounds in the body. Losing excess weight is also crucial in avoiding inflammation. Keeping estrogen and progesterone levels in check is also effective. Environ-mental toxicity and liver toxicity affects the liver's function which affects the body's ability to burn fat and eliminate toxins.

EXCESS INSULIN

Too much insulin will make you gain weight because it will store unused glucose as fat. It will also block the use of stored fat as an energy source which makes it very difficult for people to lose fat, especially around the abdominal area. Furthermore, an excess insulin level causes one to eat more because it suppresses the appetite-controlling hormone, leptin. Also, insulin causes the hormone dopamine to increase which causes the desire to eat in order to experience pleasure.
The correct amount of insulin however has huge benefits to the body. It is one of the main anabolic hormones which initiates the metabolic pathways that rebuild body proteins while preventing protein breakdown. Hence the correct levels of insulin encourage the growth of your muscles and refilling of your glycogen stores. Insulin also acts on testosterone, the male sex hormone, which is crucial for growth and muscle tissue maintenance.

Some of the main reasons for insulin overload are:
• Consuming high amounts of processed carbohydrates such as sugary drinks, sodas, foods high in fructose corn syrup, packaged low fat foods and artificial sweeteners
• Low protein intake
• Inadequate fat intake
• Deficient fiber intake
• Chronic stress
• Lack of exercise
• Over-exercising
• Steroid-based medication
• Poor liver function and high toxicity in body
• Aging

Another negative effect on men and women is the high insulin levels can increase activity of an aromatase enzyme in fat cells which causes testosterone to be converted to estrogen in men, where they deposit more fat in the female areas such as the abdominals and chest, where the chest starts to look more like breasts. Also men may start to experience a lower sex drive and erectile dysfunction. Women also get increased fat storage in the abdominals and start to have shrinking, sagging breasts, abnormal hair growth, acne and male-pattern baldness.

LOW DOPAMINE

Low levels of dopamine will affect well-being, alertness, learning, creativity, attention and concentration. Also low levels have been linked to Parkinson's disease. Low levels can cause us to crave food, sex or stimulation, however, too much can cause addictive behaviour. Therefore, dopamine is released not only during pleasurable experiences, but also during times of stress as well.

Research has shown why foods can be addictive. Addictive stimulant foods and non-foods, such as chocolate, caffeine, sugar and cigarettes, cause us to get a dopamine "rush" to overcome our fatigue.

In addition, abusive drugs, alcohol, cocaine, amphetamines and sugar can mess with our dopamine balance. For example, when people are trying to quit smoking, they tend to eat more because both food and nicotine share similar dopamine stimulating pathways.

LOW SEROTONIN

Serotonin (sometimes referred to as 5 - HT or 5-hydroxytryptamine) is a substance that occurs naturally in our body. It is a neurotransmitter that carries signals between and along nerve cells called neurons. It's found mainly in the intestines and our central nervous system (CNS), which includes your brain and your blood platelets. It regulates and affects a number of the following areas of our body functions:

This neurotransmitter is produced in your digestive tract. Low levels can affect your mood, emotions, memory and cravings for carbohydrates. The low levels can impact self-esteem, pain tolerance, sleep habits, appetite, digestion and body temperature regulation. When we are depressed, we naturally crave starches and sugars to cause serotonin levels to increase. Also when it is cold and there is less sunlight the levels decrease, hence people tend to become more depressed and eat more carbohydrates and sugars which cause weight gain.

Too much serotonin can result in life-threatening conditions such as rapid pulse, headaches, nausea, high blood pressure, decreased appetite, sweating, dilated pupils and eventually unconsciousness.

It affects our brain which affects our moods, hence it's called "feel - good" chemical.
Serotonin affects our bowel function like reducing our appetite as you eat. The platelet cells in your blood release serotonin when you have any kind of tissue damage, where vasoconstriction occurs and narrowing of the arteries causes the blood flow to slow down as part of the

blood-clotting process.

Furthermore, research has show high levels of serotonin can cause decreased bone density leading to osteoporosis. Low levels due to alcohol intoxication can increase sexual desire. But the reverse effect where from medication people's level of serotonin will be higher producing decreased levels of sexual desire.

Some of the reasons for low serotonin levels are due to the fact the body may not be producing enough or the body isn't using it efficiently because of fewer or faulty serotonin receptors absorbing serotonin too quickly.

Also, low levels of vitamin B6 and vitamin D are related to low serotonin. In addition, Tryptophan is an essential amino acid that must be obtained through food to produce serotonin. Also, many of the antidepressant medications boost serotonin levels in the brain which decreases the depression in people and improves their mood.

EXCESS CORTISOL

This is a hormone that is closely linked as an indicator of stress responses in the body. It is secreted by the adrenal glands and involved in the following functions:
- Proper glucose metabolism
- Regulation of blood pressure
- Insulin release for blood sugar maintenance
- Immune function
- Inflammatory response

While cortisol is a necessary function of the body's response to stress, it's Important that the body's relaxation response be activated so the body can return to normal. However, in many cases in our high-stress modern society the response is activated so often that the body does not have a chance to return to normal, which leads to chronic stress. Hence excess cortisol levels in the bloodstream for long periods lead to the following negative outcomes in the body:
- Impaired cognitive performance
- Suppressed thyroid function
- Blood sugar imbalances such as hyperglycemia
- Decrease bone density
- Decrease In muscle tissue
- Higher blood pressure
- Lowered immunity and inflammatory responses in the body, I.e. slow wound healing
- Increased abdominal fat, which is associated with a greater amount of health problems

than fat deposited in other areas of the body. Some of the health issues that arise from too much stomach fat are heart attacks, strokes, developing metabolic syndrome, higher levels of "bad" cholesterol (LDL) and lower levels of "good" cholesterol (HDL).

The adrenal glands produce high amounts of the hormone cortisol under situations of chronic stress, whether from physical, emotional, mental and environmental, real or imagined. Experiencing cold, hunger, low blood pressure, pain, broken bones, injuries, inflammation, sleep-wake cycle, intense exercise and emotional upsets activate the brain to pro-duce this hormone.
Furthermore, anxiety, depression, post-traumatic stress disorder or exhaustion or digestive disorder will also increase cortisol. Also, the body releases blood sugar and stored fat to provide the body with energy for a flight or fight action. However, if no physical exertion takes place then the excess sugars and fats end up increasing your waistline.

LOW DHEA

This is also produced by the adrenal glands. IT helps to make other hormones, like testosterone in men and estrogen in women. Your DHEA levels are the highest when you are a young adult. They get lower as you age. The full name of this hormone is dehydroepi-androsterone (DHEA) and it is a precursor to the sex hormones estrogen and testosterone. It helps sup- port immune system especially for preventing autoimmune imbalances, aids in tissue repair, improves sleep and counteracts negative effects of cortisol. It helps us with fat loss, gaining muscle and libido. It helps you feel motivated, youthful and energetic. Hence it is called an anti-aging hormone.

Low levels have been linked to the following conditions:
* Diabetes
* Dementia
* Increased body fat
* A decrease in muscle
* Loss of sense of well-being
* Bone density depletion
* Low libido,
* Trouble getting and keeping an erection
* Lupus
* Poor ability to handle stress
* AIDS

- Chronic fatigue syndrome

Too much DHEA can trigger excess testosterone and estrogen which leads to cancer, hair loss, anger, aggression and acne in both men and women. Women may also experience deeper voice, hair loss and abnormal growth of facial hair.

LOW GABA (GAMMA-AMINO BUTYRIC ACID)

This is an inhibitory neurotransmitter, meaning it is a brain chemical that blocks certain communication between nerve cells in brain. This brain chemical that has a calming effect on you or it can boost your mood. Therefore it decreases anxiety, muscle tension and pain. Low levels have been linked to anxiety or mood disorders, epilepsy and chronic pain. Deficient levels may be caused by inadequate nutrition, prolonged stress and genetics.
There are some natural herbs that have been found to Increase GABA levels. These are valerian, hops, chamomile, passionflower, St. John's Wort, Magnolia and Kava. They are also used to reduce anxiety, pain levels, insomnia and restlessness.

EXCESS ESTROGEN

Estrogen is mainly produced in the ovaries before menopause in females and in the adrenal glands and fat cells after menopause. Men also produce a certain amount but not have as much as women. Too much estrogen is produced in men who have high excess fat. It can in some cases cause men to take on female characteristics like enlarged nipples of their chest. This will cause the male body to convert testosterone to estrogen. Furthermore, too much estrogen and not enough can also decrease men's libido. Estradiol a predominant form of estrogen is critical in male sexual functions such as sexual desire in the brain, erectile function of the penis and sperm production.
Too much estrogen in women causes toxic fat gain, water retention and bloating. Also breast tenderness, pain or swelling can occur. Irregular menstruation can be another symptom of too much estrogen in women. It also causes the pear shaped body in premenopausal women where much of the weight is around the hips. Furthermore, many menopausal women and men end up with an apple shape where much of the fat is in the abdominal area. Here are some more additional symptoms linked to estrogen dominance in women :
- Water retention
- Brain fog
- Insomnia

- Infertility
- Fibrocystic breasts
- Uterine Fibroids

Two ways that we accumulate excess estrogen is either our body produces too much of it or we can get too much of it from our foods and the environment. Such things as the toxic pesticides, herbicides and growth hormones in our foods help to encourage more estrogen production from our fat cells.

LOW ESTROGEN

Low levels of estrogen affect the body's health negatively and its appearance. During menopause, woman find fat accumulates around their waist. Furthermore, a decrease in estrogen causes an increase in insulin. With the onset of menopause, women experience a decline in serotonin. This causes increased cravings in carbohydrates which increase insulin levels further. Also one of the symptoms that occurs after menopause is vaginal atrophy which is thinning, drying and inflammation of the vaginal walls. This causes intercourse painful and can lead to distressing urinary symptoms.

Major causes of estrogen deficiency are:
- Aging/menopause
- Premature ovarian failure
- Surgical menopause (removal of ovaries)
- Smoking
- High levels of stress
- Low-fat diets
- Exceedingly low body fat

LOW PROGESTERONE

Progesterone is produced in the ovaries before menopause and in small amounts by the adrenal glands after menopause. Progesterone levels become higher in the second half of the menstrual cycle, causing thickening of the uterine wall in preparation for the implantation of a fertilized egg. If none occurs, then the progesterone levels decline and the menstrual flow starts. Progesterone is a main hormone involved in the menstrual cycle and mainte-nance of pregnancy. It helps in breast development and breast feeding. It complements some of the effects of estrogen, another female hormone. Men produce a small amount of progesterone to help develop sperm.

Progesterone is important during childbearing years. If your progesterone levels are low then you may have trouble getting or staying pregnant. After a woman's ovaries release an egg, the progesterone levels rise to help thicken the uterine lining so the egg can implant. If the progesterone levels are low in women they can experience headaches, irregularity in menstrual cycle and mood changes, anxiety or depression.

Progesterone decline occurs because of the following:
- High stress causes body to use up progesterone to increase cortisol production.
- Lack of ovulation
- Low levels of luteinizing hormone (LH) released by brain to activate production of
- progesterone
- Hypothyroidism
- Excess Prolactin: hormone stimulates breast development during pregnancy and milk pro-duction during nursing. However, too much prolactin can suppress progesterone pro-duction.

EXCESS PROGESTERONE

Progesterone belongs to a group of steroid hormones called progestogens. Similar to es-tro-gen, progesterone has to be balanced in order to maintain a lean body. Excess proges-terone is rare, but is often seen in people who use progesterone creams or pills. Too much can cause acne, bloating, water retention, depression and weight gain. Also, if there are high levels in children, it can lead to early puberty where they will grow facial hair, experience enlargement of their penis and clitoris. A child may end up being tall but short as an adult. As adults if the levels are too high it can lead to infertility, obesity and hypertension.

LOW TESTOSTERONE

Testosterone is a major muscle building hormone, produced by the ovaries in women, in the testes in men and the adrenal glands in both males and females. It is an androgen, meaning it stimulates the development of male characteristics. It is present in greater levels in men than women. It initiates the development and is essential for the production of sperm in adult life. This hormone also signals the body to make new blood cells, ensures that muscles and bones stay strong during and after puberty and enhances libido both in men and women. It's also linked to many changes seen in boys during puberty, such as increase in height, body and pubic hair growth, enlargement of the penis, testes and prostate gland, and changes in sexual and aggressive behaviour. It also regulates the secretion of luteinizing hormone and follicle stimulating hormone. To effect these changes, testosterone is often converted into another androgen called dihydrotestosterone.

It enhances libido, bone density, muscle mass, strength, motivation, memory, fat burning and skin tone. In men it affects sperm production, causes growth of the prostate gland. It also helps in maintaining motivation and mood. Low levels have been linked to aging, obesity, osteoporosis and heart disease. Also the use of endocrine-suppressing estrogen-like compounds used in pesticides and other farming chemicals are seen as causes for the decline in testosterone in males.

Low levels in women can affect production of new blood cells, lower sex drive, weight gain and changes in mood. Long term can lead to contributing to heart disease, poor memory, and loss of bone density.

This loss can lead to andropause in men considered as male menopause. About 30% or more of males are affected. The main effects are loss in muscle mass and increase in body fat.

Some of the ways to Increase testosterone in both men and women is through eating foods high in zinc. The recommended amounts for males are 11 mg and females are 8 mg per day. The following foods have the highest amount of Zinc:

- 6 Oysters equals 26.6 mg Zinc
- Oz Tahini 2.9 mg Zinc
- Tbsp Hemp Seeds 2.97 mg Zinc
- 29 g Baking Chocolate 2.79 mg Zinc
- 309 g Lean Beef 27.13 mg Zinc
- Oz Whey Protein Isolate Oz 2.44 mg Zinc
- Oz Beef Jerky 2.30 mg Zinc
- Oz Pumpkin Seeds 2.21 mg Zinc
- Oz Sesame Seeds 2.17 mg Zinc

Furthermore, reducing sugars in the diet also Increases testosterone, because too much fructose and glucose in the body can turn off the gene that regulates testosterone and estrogen in the body. Cold Showers also enhance testosterone production because it cools the temperature of the testicles so it can produce sperm optimally. Also cold showers in-creases the over- all strength, energy levels and libido of men and estrogen levels of women which increases their sex drive as well. Alcohol consumption needs to be limited because too much can stop production of free testosterone. Eggs are the best food to increase testosterone. The saturated fat in eggs helps form free testosterone. In addition, vitamin D levels need to be optimal for the testosterone to increase. Therefore, regular exposure of the skin in the sun is Important.

Another food that is good for boosting your testosterone levels is avocados. They have 70% monounsaturated fat, 16% saturated fat and 13% polyunsatu-rated fat. They also help in preventing the conversion of testosterone into estrogen.

For serious decreases in testosterone levels, it may be helpful for testosterone replace-ment therapy with a doctor. The studies show that there is remarkable improvement in erection dysfunction, libido, muscle increase and fat loss.

HIGH TESTOSTERONE

Excess testosterone is not common in men, but is seen in about 10% of women. Usually the adrenal glands overproduce which cause polycystic ovarian syndrome (PCOS) and hirsutism (excess hair growth). It also causes acne, facial growth, male pattern hair loss, insulin resistance, irritability, anger, and decrease in breast size. Furthermore, this excess hormone activates weight gain in women, causing them to take on the apple body type.

In men, too much testosterone makes them aggressive, experience acne, increased hair loss, increased risk of prostate enlargement or cancer and increased hemoglobin. Men will increase their muscle mass but they can also decrease their sperm count due to decreased sperm production and shrunken testicles. Also high levels can occur from testicular or adrenal tumors. In addition, steroid use can also elevate high levels of testosterone. Furthermore, some males have a genetic predisposition for high levels of testosterone which makes them

a candidate for increased levels of the "bad" cholesterol which then can lead to heart issues resulting in heart attacks, cardiovascular disease, or stroke. Also, sleep apnea and infertility can result as well.

LOW THYROID HORMONE PRODUCTION (HYPOTHYROIDISM)

The thyroid gland is in the front of our neck below the Adam's apple. It produces thyroid hormones that influence every cell, tissue and organ in the body. These hormones regulate our metabolism, organ function, heart rate, cholesterol, body weight, energy, muscle contraction, relaxation, skin and hair texture. It also affects bowel function, fertility, menstrual regularity, memory, mood and other bodily processes.

Hypothyroidism is especially common in women between ages 35 and 65, about 13% of women will have an underactive thyroid. This proportion rises to 20% among women over 65. Women with low levels of thyroid hormones seem to give birth to children with lower IQs. When the hormone levels are low, it is called hypothyroidism. There are about 13 million Americans with this condition.

People suffering from hypothyroidism experience:
- Constant tiredness, less energy, sleeping a lot because of the low thyroid function
- Digestion is slow and weight gain usually occurs because your body converts fewer calories into energy, leaving more to be stored as fat.
- They also can have extremely dry skin, hair loss,
- Irregular menses, heavy menstrual bleeding,
- Poor memory, depression, decreased libido, constipation and slower mental processes.

Untreated hypothyroidism can increase your risk of high cholesterol, high blood pressure and heart disease. This can be diagnosed with a blood test and treated with medication. The symptoms can differ from person to person.

Some of the reasons for low thyroid hormone functions are:
- Pituitary or hypothalamus not sending signal to thyroid
- Low DHEA and excess cortisol inhibit thyroid function
- Toxic levels of mercury in the body
- High levels of estrogen and low progesterone
- High consumption of soy-based foods, beverages
- Pesticides in water and exposure to polybrominated biphenyls and carbohydrate disulfides
- Low levels of iodine, tyrosine and selenium

LOW ACETYLCHOLINE

Acetylcholine is the neurotransmitter that allows flow of communication between nerves and muscles. Also movement, coordination and muscle tone are influenced by the acetylcholine because it is the messenger molecule that allows the contraction of your muscles. This hormone declines as we age and could be one of the main reasons why the elderly struggle with constipation.
As we exercise we reduce the amount of acetylcholine. However, one can take natural supplements to stimulate Acetylcholine which will improve stamina and post-exercise fatigue. REM sleep, memory, mental alertness, concentration and learning are linked to acetylcholine as well. Furthermore, this decline in the hormone is linked to memory loss, depression, mood changes, insomnia and Alzheimer's disease.

LOW MELATONIN

Melatonin is the hormone released by the pineal gland to regulate our 24 hour body clock. It influences our nervous system, endocrine and immune systems. Melatonin production reaches its peak between 1 a.m. and 3 a.m. when it is quite dark. Exposure to even small amounts of light can disrupt this process. When we sleep in total darkness, melatonin is released in the body causing a slight temperature drop in the body which causes Growth Hormone to be released and allows it to do its growth and repair work. It only is in the bloodstream for 30 minutes. During this time it Induces in the liver and other cells of the body another hormone called insulin like growth factor I (IGF-I). Almost every cell in the body is affected by this hormone, especially muscle, bone, liver, kidney, skin, lung and nerve cells. Therefore, if we sleep with lights on or eat too close to bedtime, this natural cool-down will not take place causing low levels of melatonin and growth hormone. Hence you do not experience proper growth of muscle, repair and complete recuperation of the body.

In addition, you can also disrupt melatonin production if you smoke, take aspirin, ibuprofen, caffeinated products, or alcohol regularly.

Melatonin is a derivative of serotonin and is also dependent on adequate protein intake in the diet, which has tryptophan, the amino acid which is the building block of both melatonin and serotonin. Melatonin declines with age so it may be helpful to supplement for people over 45 who are having sleep challenges.

LOW GROWTH HORMONE

Growth hormone almost affects every cell in the body. It also has major effects on our feelings, actions and appearance. Since this hormone declines in the body as one ages, growth hormone supplements are often used to slow down the effects of aging. It is secreted during deep sleep and while we exercise. It's essential for tissue repair, muscle building, bone density and healthy body composition. When we sleep in total darkness, melatonin is released which cools the body. As this occurs, growth hormone is released and does its regenerative work.

If we sleep with exposure to light or eat too close to bedtime, the natural melatonin cooling process will not occur. Low melatonin and growth hormone levels affect the important role of sleep on fat loss.

Once released in the blood stream, growth hormone (GH) only has a 30 minute life span. It goes to the liver and many cells of the body to help produce another hormone called insulin-like growth factor I (IGF-I). This hormone affects muscle, bone, liver, kidney, skin, lung and nerve cells. This hormone is measured as a marker of the growth hormone production and is responsible for most of the restorative effects on the body attributed to the growth hormone (GH).

Some of the results of deficient levels of GH are:

- Premature cardiovascular disease
- Loss of bone disease
- Abdominal obesity
- Decreased muscle mass, poor posture
- Thinning or sagging skin
- Depressed mood; anxiety
- Elevated levels of LDL cholesterol
- Slow wound healing
- Fatigue
- Low stamina for exercise
- Poor immune function

Taking extra growth hormone can give benefits such as less abdominal fat, more muscle mass, fewer wrinkles, increased bone mass, improved cholesterol levels and stronger immune system function. However, there are associated risks when too much is taken. You can raise blood sugar, contribute to insulin resistance, increase risk of type 2 diabetes, and cause abnormal bone growth. Research has also shown that it can be linked to certain types of malignancies, especially prostate cancer.4

Health Results Definitions

CARDIOVASCULAR SYSTEM

We are not using this device to diagnose clients; only doctors can legally do that. We are giving our clients extra data results that will help us help them with implementing a proper nutritional program, therapy, or whatever treatment you provide as a health practitioner. If you are a medical doctor, you can use this device as an additional assessment tool along with x-rays, blood test reports, etc. to help confirm various conditions of your patients.

In this section, we will cover the main health data of the Bio-scan results in the order listed on the scan results page. We will focus on the data results that are mainly relevant from the Vital Health Nutrition Program assessments. If you offer another health modality, like acupuncture, registered massage, osteopathy, chiropractic care or naturopathic care, then your understanding of the body and health conditions should be enough to read the data shown and determine your treatment plan.

Not all the data results will be covered here, just the ones related to basic nutritional deficiencies and health issues, such as high cholesterol, liver fat content, bone mineral density, etc. These are the main conditions that can be corrected with improved lifestyle, nutrition, therapy and exercise. You can look at other systems and organs based upon a special condition the client has and look over the definition section for that data result, the hormonal assessment, health intake sheet and food score and come up with your conclusions about what the main issues and needs of your clients are.

BLOOD VISCOSITY

Blood viscosity is the thickness and stickiness of blood, and it is a direct measure of the resistance of blood to flow through vessels. Increased blood viscosity can be caused by an increase in red cell mass or increased red cell deformity, increased plasma levels of fibrinogen and coagulation factors and dehydration. The two most important determinants of blood viscosity are the hematocrit and fibrinogen levels. Hematocrit is a simple blood test done to measure the red blood cells in a person's blood. Red blood cells (erythrocytes) are important because they carry oxygen through your body. A low or high red blood cell count can indicate a medical condition or disease.

Blood can be affected by excess cholesterol, fat and toxic food which will thicken the blood and its sludge will deposit in the artery walls. When you clean eating habits, blood will clear in a number of days. Go to the definitions section and it will explain more of the health conditions associated with high blood viscosity.

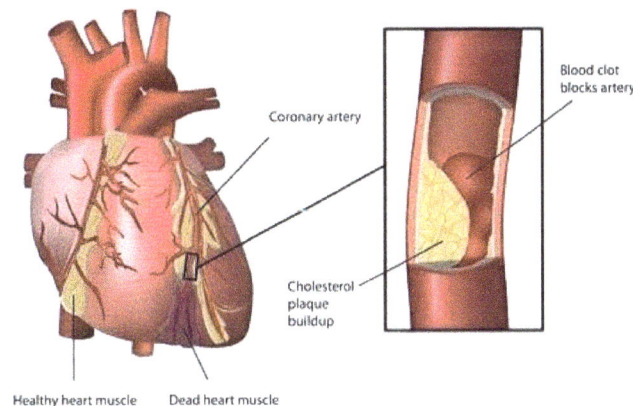

Coronary artery

Blood clot blocks artery

Cholesterol plaque buildup

Healthy heart muscle   Dead heart muscle

CHOLESTEROL CRYSTAL

This is a solid, crystalline form of cholesterol found in gallstones and arteriosclerosis. Look at the high cholesterol level indicated on the data. The high amount of cholesterol in the blood vessels can lead to arteriosclerosis, blood stagnation, major adverse cardio events and chest pain. Low levels of LDL cholesterol is rare but if it occurs there is an increased risk of cancer or hemorrhagic stroke. Symptoms of low cholesterol are hopelessness, nervousness, confusion, agitation, difficulty making a decision and changes in your mood, sleep, or eating patterns.

High cholesterol has no symptoms. Blood test is the only way to detect it. However it can lead to coronary microvascular disease. With high cholesterol you can develop fatty deposits in your blood vessels. These deposits can break suddenly and form a clot that causes a heart attack or stroke.

You can reduce Cholesterol quickly by eating mainly fruits, vegetables, whole grains and beans. Keep your fat intake small, eat more plant sources of protein and stay away from refined flour foods. Even though the amount of exercise has been a matter of debate, most health organizations recommend a minimum of 30 minutes per day of moderate to vigorous exercise, such as walking, jogging, biking, few laps at the pool, some weight-lifting and some yoga five times a week. Also some vigorous aerobic activity for at least 20 minutes three times a week. This can raise your high density lipoprotein (HDL) which is the good cholesterol. It takes about It takes about three to six months to see lower LDL numbers through diet and exercise. Usually it takes longer to see the changes in women verses men.

There are three main cholesterol levels doctors monitor: triglycerides, HDL and LDL. Exercise has the greatest effect on lowering triglycerides and increasing HDL. However, it does not have much impact on LDL unless you combine dietary change and weight loss. You also need to make sure to monitor how you feel if you have high cholesterol when exercising. If you experience chest pain, excessive shortness of breath, dizziness or lightheadedness stops immediately!

BLOOD FAT
Take note of two types of negative blood fat states in your clients. The primary hyperlipo-proteinemia is where there is too much fat in the blood due to genetic mutations, drugs and a poor diet high in fat.

The secondary hyperlipoproteinemia condition is too much fat in the blood because the body cannot break it down due to health conditions like diabetes, pancreatitis, arterioschlerosis or hypothyroidism. Too much fat in the blood can lead to fatty deposits in the blood vessels in the body, including the coronary arteries which supply the heart muscle with blood. This can lead to narrowing or hardening of the coronary arteries.

Some of the symptoms of high blood fat in the form of high levels of LDL and triglycerides can appear as chest pain (angina) or nausea and fatigue. Although you need triglycerides to supply your body with energy, having too much in your blood can Increase the risk of heart disease. About 25% of adults in the US have elevated blood triglyceride levels over 200 mg/dl. Some of the main conditions are obesity, uncontrolled diabetes, regular alcohol use and high-calorie diet.

Ways to Reduce Blood Fat

1. Decreasing calories consumed is very effective in lowering the triglyceride levels. Even after people regain lost weight, their blood triglyceride levels remained 24-26% lower.

2. Limit the amount of sugar in the diet per day including foods that convert to sugar in the body such as fruit juice, soft drinks, sweet deserts and high carbohydrate foods such as breads, pasta, white rice, etc.. The recommended amount is no more than 6 - 9 teaspoons of sugar per day in various forms.

3. Also follow a low carbohydrate diet where you consume 26% of your daily calories from low carbohydrate foods like raw vegetables, lettuce, kale, celery, cucumbers, etc. . Furthermore, this will drop the triglyceride levels.

4. Eat more foods high in fiber like fruits, vegetables, whole grains, nuts, cereals and legumes. More fiber in the diet can decrease the absorption of fats and sugar in your small Intestine, helping to lower the amount of triglycerides in your blood.

5. Aerobic Exercise done regularly increases levels of HDL cholesterol in the blood which then can lower blood triglycerides. When this is combined with a weight-loss program it's even more effective.

6. Avoid foods with Trans-fatty acids which are made partially with partially hydrogenated oils. The foods you want to avoid as much as possible are baked and fried foods. Their

7. inflammatory properties have been linked to many health problems including increased LDL levels and heart disease. It can also increase triglyceride levels. However, there are organic places that make baked breads and desserts from whole grain flour like spelt, oats and healthy oils.

8. Eat fatty fish which is high in omega-3- fatty acids which is a type of polyunsaturated fatty acid. Research has shown that consuming this regularly can decrease the risk of death from heart disease by 36%. The best sources of fish that are quite high in this omega-3 Issalmon, herring, tuna, and mackerel.

9. Increase Your Intake of Unsaturated Fats can reduce blood triglyceride levels, especially when they are replacing the bad fats. Monounsaturated and polyunsaturated fats can reduce blood triglyceride levels. Monosaturated fats are found in foods like olive oil, nuts and avocados. Polyunsaturated fats are present in vegetable oils and fatty fish. To maximize the triglyceride-lowering benefits of unsaturated fats, use cold press olive oil instead of other type of foods in your diet that contain Trans-fatty acids or highly processed vegetable oil.

10. Insulin resistance is another factor that can cause high blood triglycerides. After each meal the pancreas releases insulin into the bloodstream so it can transport glucose to our cells to be processed and used for energy. However, if there is too much insulin in your blood the body can become resistant to it so the insulin is not used effectively. This can lead to a build-

up of both glucose and triglycerides in the blood. But, by setting regular eating pattern you can help prevent insulin resistance occurring.

11. Limit Alcohol Intake because it is high in sugar and calories. If these calories remain un-used, they can be converted into triglycerides and stored in fat cells. Some studies have shown moderate to high alcohol consumption to increase blood triglyceride levels by 53%. But other research has shown light alcohol consumption has reduced the levels.

12. Add Soy Protein to Your Diet is rich in isoflavones, which are a type of plant compound with numerous health benefits. It lowers LDL cholesterol levels and triglyceride levels. A 2004 study compared how soy and animal protein affected triglycerides. After six weeks, soy protein was found to decrease triglyceride levels by 12.4% more than animal protein.

13. Eat More Tree Nuts. They provide a concentrated dose of fiber, omega-3 fatty acids and unsaturated fats, all of which work together to lower blood triglycerides. One study showed that each serving of tree nuts decreased triglycerides by 2.2 mg/dl. Be aware that nuts are high in calories. Twenty three almonds contain 163 calories so moderate portion size is important. Studies have also shown that the greatest health benefits are derived when you consume 3 - 7 servings of nuts per week.

Following Tree Nuts Are:
- Almonds
- Pecans
- Walnuts
- Cashews
- Pistachios
- Brazil Nuts
- Macadamia nuts

14. Try a Natural Supplement. Some of the herbs and supplements can also lower blood tri-glycerides.

Here are some supplements that have been confirmed by studies to work.

Fish oil - studies have shown that it can reduce triglyceride levels by 48%

Fenugreek - traditionally used to stimulate milk production in young mothers but it also has shown to be effective in reducing blood triglyceride levels.

Garlic extract - studies have shown because of its anti-inflammatory properties it can reduce triglyceride levels.

Guggul - also decreases triglyceride levels when used with nutrition therapy in patients with high cholesterol.

Curcumin - 2012 study found that supplementing with a low dose of curcumin can cause a significant drop in blood triglycerides.

VASCULAR RESISTANCE

This shows you how much resistance there is in the vessels of the circulatory system of the heart. It is the resistance that must be overcome to push blood through the circulatory system and create flow. It is used to maintain organ perfusion, the passage of fluid through the circulatory system or lymphatic system to an organ or a tissue.

In certain disease states, such as congestive heart failure, there is a hyper-adrenergic (Increased working on adrenaline (epinephrine) or noradrenaline (norepinephrine) response, causing an increase in peripheral vascular resistance. Prolonged increases in blood pressure affect several organs throughout the body. In conditions such as shock, there is a decrease in vascular resistance thus causing decreased organ perfusion which leads to organ malfunction. Peripheral vascular resistance is mediated locally by metabolites, and over a distance on a neurohormonal level, therefore, many different components may become altered leading to changes in peripheral vascular resistance.

The central dictation of peripheral vascular resistance occurs at the level of the arterioles. The arterioles dilate and constrict in response to different neuronal and hormonal signals. During an adrenergic response where norepinephrine gets released into the bloodstream, it binds to the smooth muscle cells of the vasculature binding to an alpha-1 receptor (Gq protein); this causes an increase in GTP (guanosine triphosphate involved in the peptide bond formation during protein synthesis)in the cell, which activates phospholipase C, creating IP3. IP3 signals for release of the intracellularly stored calcium as free calcium. This free calcium stimulates Calcium-dependent protein kinases into activated protein kinases which leads to contraction of the smooth muscle.[1]

VASCULAR ELASTICITY

This occurs in the arterial system where the protein elastin forms an elastic mortar between the arrays of cells that line the arteries. There, the protein provides the stability that allows the vessels to expand and contract continuously as blood pulses along.

A decrease in elasticity can indicate the arteries becoming clogged with fatty deposits (plaque), causing them to lose their elasticity and becoming narrower, therefore making the walls of the arteries thick and hard. This can cause mild arterioschlerosis, coronary heart dis- ease and even cause chest pains because of abnormal blood flow.

MYOCARDIAL BLOOD DEMAND

This is the amount of blood and oxygen required to maintain optimal function, and myo-cardial oxygen supply is the amount of oxygen provided by the blood which is controlled by the coronary arteries. Exercise strengthens the heart muscle so it becomes more efficient and better able to pump blood throughout your body. This means the heart will push out more blood with each beat, allowing it to beat slower and keep your blood pressure under control. It will also help keep the arteries and blood vessels flexible, ensuring good blood flow and normal pressure.

If its level is low, there is ineffective contraction of heart muscles and leads to coronary artery disease. Deposits of lipids, smooth muscle proliferation and endothelial dysfunction reduce the luminal diameter. Critical stenosis occurs when coronary blood flow is unable to respond to an increase in metabolic demand, usually when the diameter is reduced by 50%. Resting flow becomes affected if the diameter is reduced by 80%. . With increasing stenosis, distal arterioles dilate maximally to preserve flow up to the point where the vascular bed is maximally dilated. Further stenosis leads to a drop in flow and flow becomes pressure dependent. Flow diverted into a dilated parallel bed proximal to a stenosis is called coronary steal and can aggravate ischemia. Flow in collaterals is also often pressure dependent. Also hypertension occurs where the left ventricle undergoes hypertrophy in response to raised overload. The myofibrillar growth outstrips the capillary network, resulting in decreased capillary density. Raised intramyocardial pressure lowers the subendocardial blood flow. The pressure load increases myocardial work and oxygen demand. There is also an im-paired vasomotor response to hypoxia in hypertrophied tissue that makes it susceptible to ischaemia. Furthermore, heart failure can occur where the impaired ejection results in larger diastolic volumes, raised left ventricular stretch at the end of diastole (lVEDP) and lower coronary perfusion pressure.

This may correct itself once the client starts to exercise, lose excess fat and change their eating habits to more high anti-oxidant raw foods like fruits and vegetables.

MYOCARDIAL BLOOD PERFUSION VOLUME (MVP)

This is the volume of blood transiting through tissue at a certain rate. It can be quantified in ml/min per gram tissue when the MVP is normalized to blood pool. If the reading is high, it can mean high damage to heart. If low, it means no damage to heart but the heart may be at risk of damage. If the client has heart complications then please do not try to give any advice or recommendations, unless you are a doctor. Refer them to their doctor.

MYOCARDIAL OXYGEN CONSUMPTION (MOC)

This is the amount of oxygen that the heart requires to maintain optimal function, and the myocardial oxygen supply is the amount of oxygen provided to the heart as it is controlled by the coronary arteries.

The rates of oxygen uptake during exercise will depend on gait, economy of locomotion, body mass, and other factors. The maximal rate of oxygen uptake is the gold standard measurement for aerobic capacity. It is primarily limited by the maximal heart rate and cardiacstroke volume during exercise.

Increased heart rates that occur and longer heart contraction times cause an increase in MOC. The readings will probably be low for clients who have some sort of coronary heart disease. This is where once you help a client to start to exercise and improve their diet; the readings may increase over time.

However, a healthy client who exercises and does a lot of cardio training will probably have high readings or close to normal readings.

STROKE VOLUME
This is blood volume output per heart beat. It is the volume of blood pumped out of the left ventricle of the heart during each systolic cardiac contraction. If it is too high, it can damage the heart and a stroke can occur. If it is too low, then not enough blood is going to the heart which can also create complications. Refer the client to their doctor if they have reading that is too high or too low.

LEFT VENTRICULAR EJECTION IMPEDANCE
The resistance as the left ventricle pumps blood to the tissues cannot be too high or too low. If it is too high, it can damage the heart and a stroke can occur. If it is too low, then not enough blood is going to the heart which can also create complications. Refer the client to their doctor if they have reading that is too high or too low.

LEFT VENTRICULAR EFFECTIVE PUMP POWER

This is the effective rate at which the left ventricle performs work as the continuous product of aortic flow and ventricular pressure. The left ventricle is larger than the other chambers and essential for normal function because it provides most of the heart's pumping power. This is the contraction strength of an effective stroke of blood to the left ventricle. If the readings for this are too high it can damage the heart and a stroke can occur. If it is too low, then not enough blood is going to the heart which can also create complications. Refer the client to their doctor if they have a reading that is too high or too low..

CORONARY ARTERY ELASTICITY
The arteries leading to the heart are smooth and elastic, lined with cells called endothelium. If the reading is high, this means the vessels may have plaque build-up in their inner walls which makes them stiff and narrow. This weakened elasticity slows blood flow to the heart

muscle so it doesn't get the oxygen it needs. Also the plaque can break off, which will lead to heart failure and stroke. If the reading is too low meaning the vessels have become weak, then it can lead to dizziness, weakness and fainting. Again, if the readings of your client are very high or very low, refer them to their doctor. However, helping them with an improved diet of good fats, such as salmon, avocado and nuts, and having them start a mild exercise program, could make a positive difference in their heart issue.

CORONARY PERFUSION PRESSURE
This is the pressure of the coronary artery in blood supply to the heart. It is influenced by diastolic pressure (blood going into the coronary arteries during perfusion) and left atria pressure. If the readings are high, it indicates that the vessels have become less elastic which can lead to a risk for strokes, heart attacks, heart failure and renal failure (kidney failure).
If the readings are low, it indicates that the vessels have become weak and can cause light headedness, dizziness, weakness, fainting and in extreme cases shock. Again, this is prob-ably due to high plaque build-up in the arteries. A change in nutrition and a proper exercise program could make a hugedifference.

CEREBRAL BLOOD VESSEL ELASTICITY
The brain artery or the neck artery controlling the brain can have lesions, which leads to disorder of intracranial blood circulation and damage of brain tissue. The elasticity of hardened brain blood vessels is weakened, and the vessel cavity is narrowed, so it is easy to form cerebral thrombosis. When people with cerebral arteriosclerosis excessively drink alcohol, the blood pressure will be suddenly elevated; the blood vessels will rupture, so it is prone to form cerebral hemorrhage. If they binge drink, the concentration of alcohol in blood can reach its peak in a half hour. The alcohol can not only directly stimulate the blood vessel wall to make it lose its elasticity but also stimulate the liver to promote the synthesis of cholesterol and triglyceride, thus leading to arterioschlerosis and cerebral arterioschlerosis.
Cerebrovascular disease can be divided into acute cerebrovascular disease and chronic cerebrovascular disease according to their process. The acute cerebrovascular disease includes transient ischemic at- tack, cerebral thrombosis, cerebral embolism, hypertensive encephalopathy, cerebral hemor- rhage, sub-arachnoid hemorrhage, etc. The chronic cerebrovascular disease includes cerebral arterio-sclerosis, cerebrovascular dementia, cerebral artery steal syndrome, Parkinson's dis- ease, etc. The Cerebrovascular disease which is known generally refers to the acute cerebro- vascular disease. The chronic cerebrovascular disease is easy to be ignored by people due to it gradually taking time to develop.
The wall of the artery is made up of layers; two of them being muscle tissue and elastic tissue. When a part of the blood vessel wall weakens, it can inflate out like a balloon to form a sac-like structure.

If the Cerebral Blood Vessel Elasticity readings are high, this means that the blood vessels have lost elasticity, which can possibly lead to a risk for aneurysm (blood vessel swelling). If the Cerebral Blood Vessel Elasticity readings are low, the vessels have become weak and can cause light headedness, dizziness, weakness and even fainting.

A healthier diet of raw foods high in antioxidants can help strengthen the blood vessel walls because there are hundreds of natural phytochemicals in raw vegetables and fruits that help regenerate the body. Also, consuming lots of fresh vegetable juices done in a juicer can have a huge impact on restoring and decreasing the plaque buildup in the whole artery and vessels of the cardiovascular system. I personally have seen clients decrease their cholesterol count after doing a juice cleanse program outlined in the Vital Health Nutrition book.

GASTROINTESTINAL FUNCTION

PEPSIN SECRETION COEFFICIENT

Pepsin is a stomach enzyme that serves to digest proteins found in ingested food. Gastric chief cells secrete pepsin as an inactive zymogen called pepsinogen. Arietal cells within the stomach lining secrete hydrochloric acid that lowers the PH of the stomach. Once the PH is 1.5 to 2, it activates pepsin. If this digestive enzyme in the stomach is low, then it can mean not enough hydrochloric acid is being produced in the stomach, which means the client is not breaking down protein well. If the readings are too high, it can cause irritation to the stomach lining.

If a client has a low pepsin reading and you know by their food score results and health conditions that they suffer from weak digestion issues, a good recommendation is to have them eat more raw vegetables to help them digest protein better in the stomach. The extra enzymes of the raw vegetables and fruit juices can make a difference in these cases.

GASTRIC PERISTALSIS FUNCTION COEFFICIENT

This is where the oblique, circular and longitudinal smooth muscles on the gastric wall, and their contraction and relaxation make the stomach have the capability of peristalsis. Gastric peristalsis grinds the food for further processing as well as the role of gastric juice to make food into gruel kind of chime, and then the chime are ejected in the small intestines in batches through the pylorus. The time of processing food in the stomach is different. The processing time of carbohydrate foods is shorter than that of protein foods, and longer for fats and oils. Hence, we are not hungry after eating meats and oily foods. The food is preliminarily digested by the gastric motion (peristalsis) and gastric juice (mucus, gastric acid, protease, etc.) secreted by the stomach to form a paste (chyme), and then enters the small intestines (including: duodenum, jejunum, and ileum) after eating about 3-4 hours.

A low reading can indicate the client has poor nutrition, not enough fiber, not enough ex-ercise and is not drinking enough water. Eating more raw vegetables and whole grains can increase the peristalsis action in a person's digestion.5

GASTRIC FUNCTION ABSORPTION COEFFICIENT
The gastric gland in gastric mucosa secretes a kind of colorless and transparent acidic gastric juice, and the gastric gland of an adult can secrete 1.5-2.5 liters of gastric juice each day. Gastric juice contains three main components, namely, pepsin, hydrochloric acid and mucus. The pepsin can decompose proteins in food into proteose and protease with smaller molecules. Hydrochloric acid is gastric acid. Gastric acid can change protease with no activity into active pepsin and create a suitable acidic environment for pepsin, having the function for killing bacteria entering into the stomach with food. Gastric acid can stimulate the secretion of pancreatic juice, bile and small intestinal fluid entering into the small intestines. The acidic environment caused by the gastric acid can help the small intestines absorb iron and calcium. With the role of lubrication, gastric mucus can reduce the damage of food, for gastric mucosa can also reduce the erosion of gastric acid and pepsin, having a protective effect of the stomach.
A high reading can indicate that the client may have acid indigestion and a low reading can mean low absorption of proteins from the foods being digested in the stomach.

SMALL INTESTINE PERISTALSIS FUNCTION COEFFICIENT
Small intestine peristalsis is in a unique movement style, being an alternating motion of rhythmic contraction and relaxation with circular muscle of the intestine as the main mover. Function: it promotes chyme and digestive juice to be fully mixed for chemical digestion; it makes chyme close to the intestine wall to promote absorption; it squeezes the intestine wall to promote reflux of blood and lymph. Once past the stomach, a typical peristaltic wave only lasts for a few seconds, traveling at only a few centimeters per second. Its primary purpose is to mix the chyme in the intestine rather than to move it forward in the intestine
Many of the clients you assess will show a low peristalsis reading of the small intestine. This usually indicates slow digestion, bloating and constipation.

SMALL INTESTINE ABSORPTION FUNCTION COEFFICIENT
The small intestine is the part of the intestines where 90% of the digestion and absorption of food occurs, the other 10% taking place in the stomach and large intestine. The main function of the small intestine is absorption of nutrients and minerals from food.
In the intestine the absorption of sugar: the sugar is generally decomposed into simple sugar to be absorbed, and only a small amount is absorbed.
The absorption of protein: 50-100 grams of amino acids and a small amount of dipeptides and tripeptides are absorbed each day.

The absorption of fat: mixed small micelles are transported to arrive in the microvilli, bile salts remain in the intestine, and fat digestion products (fatty acids, monoglyceride, cholesterol and lysolecithin) are diffused into the cells. The middle and short-chain fatty acids (<10-12c) do not need to be esterified, and can be directly diffused into the capillaries of the villi. Other fat digestion products are esterified in smooth endoplasmic reticulum to form triglycerides (long-chain fatty acids + glyceride), cholesterol ester and lecithin to combine with the apo-protein / apolipoprotein (synthesized by intestinal epithelial cells) into chylomicrons; the chylomicrons are packaged into secretory granules in the GC for exocytosis to enter into the thoracic duct, then are absorbed by the lymphatic vessel and finally enter the blood circulation.

The absorption of water: the water is passively absorbed by osmotic pressure gradient formed by the absorption of nutrients and electrolytes in the intestine (osmosis).

Usually the readings in many of the clients will be low in this section particularly in people who eat foods that are high density, low water content and low enzymes. These foods are common especially in a western culture. The absorption rate will be slow due to the quality of the foods being low. Therefore, if there is refined sugar and preservatives in the food there can also be inflammation as well occurring in the small intestine.

LIVER FUNCTION

The liver's main job is to filter the blood coming from the digestive tract, before passing it to the rest of the body. The liver also detoxifies chemicals and metabolizes drugs. As it does so, the liver secretes bile that ends up back in the intestines.

There are five main functions of the liver:
• Bile production and excretion.
• Excretion of bilirubin, cholesterol, hormones, and drugs.
• Metabolism of fats, proteins, and carbohydrates.
• Enzyme activation.
• Storage of glycogen, vitamins, and minerals.
• Synthesis of plasma proteins, such as albumin, and clotting factors

PROTEIN METABOLISM
The liver also plays an important role in the metabolism of proteins: liver cells change amino acids in foods so that they can be used to produce energy, or make carbohydrates or fats. A toxic substance called ammonia is a by-product of this process.

Protein in food is digested and absorbed by the intestinal tract to be sent to the liver for conversion and reorganization, different types of amino acids are metabolized to manufacture a variety of proteins for the cell's needs according to the body's need. In addition, the liver will decompose the useless protein into amino acids, and then the amino acids are further changed into urea to be excreted by the kidney or intestinal tract.

In many cases, you will have low readings in this section, meaning that either the liver is not functioning well or the foods which are processed are too high in fat, causing higher toxicity in the liver which can contribute to the liver malfunctioning.

ENERGY PRODUCTION FUNCTION

It is also one of the organs that break down old or damaged blood cells. The liver plays a central role in all metabolic processes in the body. In fat metabolism the liver cells break down fats and pro-duce energy.

After carbohydrates are digested, the liver will carry out sugar metabolism to produce energy for the need of cells and then convert excess sugar into glycogen for storage. After fatty foods are digested, the liver will further convert fat into energy.

The readings in this section may be low because the client has not consumed enough car-bo-hydrates in their diet. The readings in the liver function will change over time as the person changes their eating habits or consumes more or less protein, fats and carbohydrates which will give different readings here. However, the low readings of this section can be used to make suggestions to your client for consuming proper amounts of healthy carbohydrates and protein. Following proper food combining principles will help them not to overwork the liver's function.

DETOXIFICATION FUNCTION

Food will produce some toxins in the digestive process and the metabolism process. The liver as well as detoxifying enzymes carry out detoxification to decompose the hazardous substances (alcohol and ammonia) into harmless substances (such as urea, water and carbo-hydrate dioxide) to be excreted out of the body. The liver plays several roles in detoxification: it filters the blood to remove large toxins, synthesizes and secretes bile full of cholesterol and other fat-soluble toxins, and enzymatically disassembles unwanted chemicals.

If this reading is high, you may want to recommend your client improve their diet, reducing alcohol consumption and processed foods, which both stress the liver's detoxification func-tion. Eventually, the liver can breakdown from high amounts of alcohol consumption, which is what, happens to alcoholics.

A low reading is not good either because it means the liver is not getting rid of the toxins fast enough; hence further health issues can occur.

BILE SECRETION FUNCTION

Bile is the end product of metabolism in the liver, which has the role of fat digestion and promotes the body to absorb fat-soluble vitamins A, D, E and K. The excess bile will be sent to gallbladder for standby. Bile is a fluid that is made and released by the liver and stored in the gallbladder. Bile helps with digestion. It breaks down fats into fatty acids, which can be taken into the body by the digestive tract.

A high reading means too much bile is being secreted which causes the gallbladder to stop functioning temporarily. This then leads to formation of gallstones. Therefore, if you have a client who already has passed gall stones and their diet is poor, you may want to suggest they follow a lower fat diet so their gallbladder does not shut down too much, creating more stones in their gallbladder.

A low reading means not enough bile is being secreted to look after digestion of fat which can lead to higher cholesterol. You may suggest, if you are looking at nutrition with a client, that they start consuming raw vegetable juice, with some black radish in the juice. The black radish stimulates the gallbladder to produce more bile which can help in digesting fat in the diet, therefore decreasing bad LDL cholesterol levels.

LIVER FAT CONTENT

If the liver fat content is more than 5% of wet weight or over 1 / 3 liver cells of per unit area on liver biopsy have lipid droplets under a microscope, the liver is called as a fatty liver. The fatty liver is also known as liver fatty degeneration which refers to fat ac-cumulation in liver cells due to a variety of causes. When a healthy person takes in meals with reasonable ingredients, the liver fat content accounts for 5% of the weight of liver. B-US can detect the fatty liver with over 30% of liver fat content.

The fatty liver is divided into obese fatty liver, alcoholic fatty liver, diabetes fatty liver which are the three common causes of fatty liver. In addition, there are nutritional disorder fatty liver, drug-induced fatty liver, acute fatty liver of pregnancy and so on. What are the symptoms of fatty liver? The person with mild fatty liver can have no discomfort. The patients with moderate or severe fatty liver can have loss of appetite, fatigue, nausea, vomiting, abdominal distension, diarrhea, liver pain, left shoulder and back pain, swollen and other symptoms. The hepatomegaly can be found by a medical examination, and a few livers have mild jaundice and spider angioma. Abnormal liver function, triglycerides and cholesterol increase can be found by a laboratory test. Early diagnosis and prompt treatment can effectively control the further development of fatty liver, so fat deposition in the liver can fade.

If the reading is high in the liver fat content, then a diet low in fat is necessary for the client. Also a weight loss program should be implemented if the client is heavy. A cleanse will also bring the fat down in the body and in the liver as well.

Helping people rebuild from the inside out.

GALLBLADDER FUNCTION

The gallbladder is a pear-shaped, hollow structure located under the liver and on the right side of the abdomen. Its primary function is to store and concentrate bile, a yellow-brown digestive enzyme produced by the liver. The gallbladder is part of the billiary tract.

SERUM GLOBULIN

Medical Definition of serum globulin. : a globulin or mixture of globulins occurring in blood serum and containing most of the antibodies of the blood.
Clients, who have compromised health, smoke and drink regularly may show low readings in their serum globulin.

TOTAL BILIRUBIN

This is a blood test that measures the amount of bilirubin in the blood because if there is a high level, it may be a sign of liver disease.
Bilirubin is a yellowish substance in your blood. It forms after red blood cells break down, and it travels through your liver, gallbladder, and digestive tract before being excreted. Typically, bilirubin levels fall somewhere between 0.3 and 1.2 milligrams per deciliter (mg/dL). Anything above 1.2 mg/dL is usually considered high. The condition of having high bilirubin levels is called hyperbilirubinemia. It's usually a sign of an underlying condition, so it's important to follow up with a doctor if test results show you have high bilirubin. Many babies are also born with high bilirubin, causing a condition called newborn jaundice. This causes yellow-tinted skin and eyes. It happens because, at birth, the liver often isn't yet fully able to process bilirubin. This is a temporary condition that usually resolves on its own within a few weeks.

ALKALINE PHOSPHATASE

Alkaline Phosphatase (ALP) is an enzyme found in several tissues throughout the body. The ALP in blood samples of healthy adults comes mainly from the liver, with most of the rest coming from bones (skeleton). Elevated levels of ALP in the blood are most commonly caused by liver disease, bile duct obstruction, gallbladder disease, or bone disorders. This test measures the level of ALP in the blood. (https://labtestsonline.org/tests/alkaline-phosphatase-alp)

SERUM TOTAL BILE ACID

Total bile acids are metabolized in the liver and can serve as a marker for normal liver function. Increases in serum bile acids are seen in patients with acute hepatitis, chronic hepatitis, liver sclerosis, and liver cancer.

A low reading indicates your client's immune system is low and the liver and gallbladder may be breaking down towards a disease. A proper 5 phase cleanse starting with a semi-juice cleanse meal plan can really help people restore and strengthen their liver and gallbladder. If there are any low or high readings for Alkaline Phosphatase and Serum Total Bile Acid, then the client may be headed towards some of the health issues outlined in the definition section of the data results of the scan.

INSULIN

Insulin is a hormone made by the pancreas that allows your body to use sugar (glucose) from carbohydrates in the food that you eat for energy or to store glucose for future use. Insulin helps keeps your blood sugar level from getting too high (hyperglycemia) or too low (hypo-glycemia).

The cells in your body need sugar for energy. However, sugar cannot go into most of your cells directly. After you eat food and your blood sugar level rises, cells in your pancreas (known as beta cells) are signaled to release insulin into your blood-stream. Insulin then attaches to and signals cells to absorb sugar from the bloodstream. Insulin is often described as a "key," which unlocks the cell to allow sugar to enter the cell and be used for energy.

High readings of insulin can signal heart problems. With proper nutritional changes, cleanses, weight-loss and exercise your client can greatly correct their heart problems in a lot of the cases. A Chinese assessment can be done where there are Chinese herbal formula supplements that help strengthen the heart. Low readings usually indicate your client is possibly on their way to becoming a diabetic. Look at all the other assessment results, such as the food score and the hormone assessment sheet, to confirm your conclusion. If you see that the client eats a lot of sugar, refined high carbohydrate foods and they are overweight, then they may well be on their way to becoming a type 2 diabetic.

PANCREATIC POLYPEPTIDE (PP)

Pancreatic polypeptide (PP) is a peptide hormone found in the islets of Langerhans and between the acinar cells that inhibits pancreatic secretion of fluid, bicarbohydrate, and enzymes. It also stimulates the gastric juice secretion, but inhibits the gastric secretion induced by pentagastrine.

High and low readings can result in various health conditions for your client. Refer here to the definition section of the data results. The results of the pancreatic polypeptide are closely tied to diabetic conditions as well. Therefore, the nutritional changes that can help diabetics can also help the negative conditions represented by the high and low readings of the PP levels.

GLUCAGON

A hormone formed in the pancreas which promotes the breakdown of glycogen to glucose in the liver. It is synthesized and secreted by pancreatic 5-cells, when the blood sugar concentration is elevated. Insulin and glucagon are vital for maintaining normal ranges of blood sugar. Insulin allows the cells to absorb glucose from the blood, while glucagon triggers a release of stored glucose from the liver.

This hormone works with insulin to keep the glucose levels in balance in the blood. Therefore, when the glucagon levels are high or low serious health conditions can occur. Please refer to the definition section of the book for this hormone result.

KIDNEY FUNCTION

Major function of the kidneys is to remove waste products and excess fluid from the body. These waste products and excess fluid are removed through the urine. The production of urine involves highly complex steps of excretion and re-absorption.

UROBILINOGEN

Urobilinogen is formed from the reduction of bilirubin. It is formed in the intestines by bacterial action. Some urobilinogen is reabsorbed, taken up into the circulation and excreted
by the kidney. Most of urobilinogen will be excreted along with feces, and other part will be absorbed by the liver back to the intestinal, then from the liver enter into the kidney or the blood and excreted out together with the urine.

URIC ACID

Uric acid is a natural waste product from the digestion of foods that contain purines. Purines are found in high levels in some foods such as: certain meats, sardines, dried beans and beer. In human blood plasma, the reference range of uric acid is between 3.6 mg/dl (~214 ?mol/l) and 8.3 mg/dl (~494 ?mol/l) (1 mg/dl=59.48 ?mol/l).[this range is considered normal by the American Medical Association manual. Uric acid concentrations in blood plasma above and below the normal range are known, respectively, as hyperuricemia and hypouricemia. Most uric acid dissolves in blood and travels to the kidneys, where it passes out in urine. Some people develop gout, kidney stones or kidney failure due to high uric acid levels. A high uric acid level may appear prior to the development of high blood pressure, heart disease or chronic kidney disease.

BLOOD UREA NITROGEN

Blood urea nitrogen (bun) measures the amount of urea nitrogen, a waste product of protein metabolism, in the blood. Urea is formed by the liver and carried by the blood to the kidneys for excretion. The amino acid deamination produces nh3 and c02, and which synthesis to urea in the liver per gram of protein metabolism of urea is 0.3g. The nitrogen has almost half content of 28/26 in the urea. Diseased or damaged kidneys cause an elevated bun because the kidneys are less able to clear urea from the bloodstream. In conditions in which renal perfusion is decreased, such as hypovolemic shock or congestive heart failure, bun levels rise.

Positive levels of both Uric Acid and Urobilinogen lead to severe health issues. Please refer to the kidney section of the definition section. For most people who are relatively healthy, check to see that these levels are normal.

PROTEINURIA

Proteinuria is increased levels of protein in the urine. This condition can be a sign of kidney damage. Proteins – which help build muscle and bone, regulate the amount of fluid in blood, combat infection and repair tissue – should remain in the blood.

There always will be a certain amount of protein essential for human life activities in the blood. A part of proteins will be filtered by sphere in the kidney and enter into the urine, but it may be absorbed in the renal tubules back to the blood. Therefore, if the function of the kidneys is normal, the protein in the urine just has a little. However, when the kidneys and catherter leakage arises obstacles that will have a large amount of protein become proteinuria. It's normal that have trace protein in a healthy person's urine, and the normal range defined as negative. When the protein in urine goes up to more than 0.15g/24h, it is called proteinuria, and this can be positive qualitative urine.

LUNG FUNCTION

Every cell in your body needs oxygen in order to live. The air we breathe contains oxygen and other gases. Once in the lungs, oxygen is moved into the bloodstream and carried through your body. At each cell in your body, oxygen is exchanged for a waste gas called carbohydrate dioxide. Your bloodstream then carries this waste gas back to the lungs where it is removed from the bloodstream and then exhaled. Your lungs and respiratory system automatically perform this vital process, called gas exchange.

In addition to gas exchange, your respiratory system performs other roles important to breathing. These include:

• Bringing air to the proper body temperature and moisturizing it to the right humidity level.

• Protecting your body from harmful substances. This is done by coughing, sneezing, filtering or swallowing them.

• Supporting your sense of smell.

VITAL CAPACITY

The volume of air occupying the lungs at different phases of the respiratory cycle subdivides into four volumes and four capacities. The four lung volumes are inspiratory reserve volume (IRV), expiratory reserve volume (ERV), tidal volume (V), and residual volume (RV), while the four lung capacities include total lung capacity (TLC), vital capacity (VC), inspiratory capacity (IC), and functional residual capacity (FRC).

Vital capacity (VC) refers to the maximal volume of air that can be expired following maximum in-spiration. It is the total of tidal volume, inspiratory reserve volume, and expiratory reserve volume (VC = V + IRV + ERV).[2] Vital capacity may be measured as inspiratory vital capacity (IVC), slow vital capacity (SVC), or forced vital capacity (FVC). The FVC is similar to VC, but it is measured as the patient exhales with maximum speed and effort.

Issues of Concern

The vital capacity can be measured using a wet or regular Spirometer. The vital capacity of a typical adult is between 3 and 5 liters. Factors that affect a person's vital capacity include age, sex, height, weight, and ethnicity. For instance, the residual volume and the functional residual capacity increase with age, resulting in a decrease in the vital capacity. Vital capacity has been found to increase with an increase in the height of a person, whereas, an increasing body mass index (BMI) is shown to correlate with a lower vital capacity.

The Vital Capacity readings indicate what the normal range should be for a fairly healthy lung condition. When the readings fall below 3348 or are higher than 3529 then the lungs of

your client are on their way to some health issues, as indicated in the definition section of the book. In one instance, I had a client who I was training and implementing some nutrition programs. He had lower than normal readings for his lungs. He had all the signs of early stage pulmonary emphysema and mild bronchitis and lung cough. He smoked half a pack a day and had quite a toxic diet for years before he came to see me.

TOTAL LUNG CAPACITY

Total lung capacity (TLC) is the amount of air the lung can contain at the height of maximum inspiratory effort. All other lung volumes are natural subdivisions of TLC. • Residual volume (RV) is the amount of air remaining within the lung after maximum exhalation.

For Total Lung Capacity, if the readings are higher than 4782 and lower than 4301, similar health conditions as indicated for low and high readings of Vital Capacity can occur in regards to the lungs of your client.

If your client smokes, it is advisable to encourage them to stop and also do a cleanse to rid their body of excess mucus in the lungs. This will also rid toxins which have accumulated in their body over the years from the various chemicals in the cigarettes.

AIRWAY RESISTANCE

Airway resistance is defined as the change in transpulmonary pressure (proximal airway pressure minus the alveolar pressure) required producing a unit flow of gas through the airways of the lung.

For airway resistance, if the readings are higher than 1,709 and lower than 1,374 bronchial asthma and similar lung diseases, as mentioned in the earlier readings, can occur.

ARTERIAL OXYGEN CONTENT PaCO2

This is the content (or concentration) of oxygen in arterial blood (Ca02) is expressed in ml of oxygen per 100 ml. Normal arterial oxygen is approximately 75 to 100 millimeters of mercury (mm Hg). Values under 60 mm Hg usually indicate the need for supplemental oxygen. Normal pulse oximeter readings usually range from 95 to 100 percent. Values under 90 percent are considered low.

For the Arterial Oxygen Content readings, if it is greater or lower than the indicated normal readings, lung weakness, bronchitis and whopping cough may develop.

BRAIN NERVE FUNCTION

The brain controls what we think and feel, how we learn and remember, and the way we move and talk. But it also controls things we're less aware of — like the beating of our hearts a

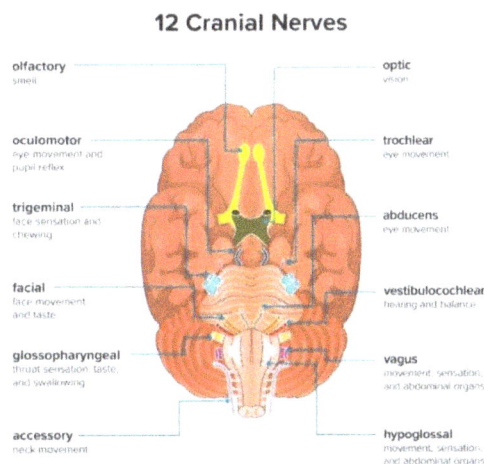

12 Cranial Nerves

olfactory
smell

optic
vision

oculomotor
eye movement and
pupil reflex

trochlear
eye movement

trigeminal
face sensation and
chewing

abducens
eye movement

facial
face movement
and taste

vestibulocochlear
hearing and balance

glossopharyngeal
throat sensation, taste,
and swallowing

vagus
movement, sensation,
and abdominal organs

accessory
neck movement

hypoglossal
movement, sensation,
and abdominal organs

the digestion of our food. Think of the brain as a central computer that controls all the body's functions. The rest of the nervous system is like a network that relays messages back and forth from the brain to different parts of the body. It does this via the spinal cord, which runs from the brain down through the back. It contains threadlike nerves that branch out to every organ and body part.

When a message comes into the brain from anywhere in the body, the brain tells the body how to react. For example, if you touch a hot stove, the nerves in your skin shoot a message of pain to your brain. The brain then sends a message back telling the muscles in your hand to pull away. Luckily, this neurological relay race happens in an instant.

STATUS OF BRAIN TISSUE BLOOD SUPPLY

The brain receives blood from two sources: the internal carotid arteries, which arise at the point in the neck where the common carotid arteries bifurcate, and the vertebral arteries. The internal carotid arteries branch to form two major cerebral arteries, the anterior and middle cerebral arteries. The right and left vertebral arteries come together at the level of the pons on the ventral surface of the brainstem to form the midline basilar artery. The basilar artery joins the blood supply from the internal carotids in an arterial ring at the base of the brain (in the vicinity of the hypothalamus and cerebral peduncles) called the circle of willis. The posterior cerebral arteries arise at this confluence, as do two small bridging arteries, the anterior and posterior communicating arteries. Conjoining the two major sources of cerebral vascular supply via the circle of willis presumably improves the chances of any region of the brain continuing to receive blood if one of the major arteries becomes occluded.

Cerebral microcirculation usually refers to the blood vessels with the diameter <150 (m, including small arteries, capillaries and small veins. However, the definition of the microcirculation has not been widely accepted, and it is not clear whether the small arteries (based on anatomical criteria, the lumen diameter > 150 (m) belong to the microcirculation. Therefore, it is defined in accordance with the vascular physiology, namely the response of a single vessel to elevated pressure inside the lumen, rather than in accordance with the diameter or structure. According to this definition, all those arteries whose lumen diameter has myogenic contractile responses to elevated pressure, and capillaries and small veins will be included in the microcirculation. The primary function of microcirculation is to make the supply of nutrients and oxygen in tissues change following with the change in demand; the second important role is to avoid the drastic fluctuation of hydrostatic pressure in capillaries to as they exchange through the barrier of capillaries; and finally, the hydrostatic pressure is significantly reduced in the microcirculation level. Thus, microcirculation has an extremely important role in deter-mining the total peripheral resistance. In addition, the microcirculation is also the first diseased parts of cardiovascular disease, in particular in the inflammatory process.

CEREBRAL ARTERIOSCEROSIS

Cerebral arteriosclerosis is the result of thickening and hardening of the walls of the arteries in the brain. Symptoms of cerebral arteriosclerosis include headache, facial pain, and impaired vision. Cerebral arteriosclerosis can cause serious health problems.

With cerebral arteriosclerosis, a variety of arterial inflammation, trauma and local cerebral vascular diseases are caused. Also such physical factors like blood diseases, the resistance of blood flow becoming greater can lead to the occurrence of ischemic cerebrovascular diseases. Transient ischemic attack whose disease causes are related to cerebral arteriosclerosis is the function disturbance caused by transient, ischemic and focal brain tissue damage. Cerebral thrombosis is mostly caused by the blocking of formed blood clots. Cerebral embolism can be induced by the fact that emboli resulting from a variety of diseases enter into the blood to block the blood vessels in the brain. In clinic, heart diseases are the most common cause; the other causes include fat in the blood after fractures, or trauma; bacterial infection; the air in the blood of pneumothorax and others, emboli formed from phlebitis and other factors block the brain blood vessels. The vessels in the brain surface are ruptured leading to cerebral hemorrhage, and cerebral hemorrhage caused by ruptured blood vessels in results in hemorrhagic cerebrovascular disease.

You want to check this section if you have a client who has heart issues, high cholesterol or had a stroke in the past. Sometimes the arteries in the brain may be thickening and getting too hard which can result in aneurysms or bleeding of the artery wall. You want to look at the readings of the Cerebral Arterioschlerosis to make sure readings are not higher than the normal.

FUNCTIONAL STATUS OF CRANIAL NERVE

The cranial nerves are a set of twelve nerves that originate in the brain. Each has a different function for sense or movement. The functions of the cranial nerves are sensory, motor, or both: sensory cranial nerves help a person to see, smell, and hear.

Cranial nerve system can be divided into three parts according to functions. The first part, which introduces the information out of the body to the brain, is called the sensory nervous system. The second part, which carries out processing and storage and drives the body to respond, is called the central nervous system, namely the majority of the brain. The third part, which drives the muscles, internal organs and glands, is called the motor nervous system which implements the decision in the brain. The third part also includes the main nervous system.

The communication among the nerve cells of the three parts depends on two factors: one is the connection networks among cranial nerve cells. The cranial nerve system has about 100 billion cranial nerve cells, and almost each person has the same number. The number of connection networks among cranial nerve cells determines whether the person is smarter than others. Each cranial nerve cell is connected with 1000-200,000 other cranial nerve cells, averaging 15,000. The other cells are neurotransmitters. Message transmission in a cranial nerve cell depends on the electrical guidance line, but message transmission between two cranial nerve cells depends on some biological or chemical substances manufactured by the body, which are called neurotransmitters. A cranial nerve cell releases a kind of neurotransmitter at the gap of the connection between it and other cranial nerve cells, and the 15000 linked cranial nerve cells produce the relevant electric guidance lines after receiving the neurotransmitter. The procedure is repeated, and the 15000 linked cranial nerve cells send the message to other 15000 linked cranial nerve cells to constantly continue. Now, there are 80 kinds of these neurotransmitters, while there are only 8-9 kinds of the main neurotransmitters. These neurotransmitters drive the various parts of the body to maintain or change their status, and are also the determinants of our sentiment.

SENTIMENT INDEX

Sentiment is people's experience of attitude toward the objective things, and the re-flection whether people's needs are satisfied. Sentiment is divided into two kinds: positive sentiment and negative sentiment. The positive sentiment can enhance immune function and promote health, therefore improving quality of life; the negative sentiment including upset, sadness, anxiety, resentment, apathy, etc., is harmful for physical and mental health. Physiological and life practice show that the bad sentiment can induce production of disease and aggravate the disease, and it can also reduce the effect of drug treatment. Because physical condition deteriorates in the elderly and the ability to resist disease-causing factors in and out of the body is reduced, the elderly is susceptible to various diseases. The common diseases include high blood pressure, heart disease, ulcer, diabetes, cancer, etc. Because of many diseases, unhealthy conditions and even the threat of death, the elderly is prone to negative sentiment and pessimistic minds and is demoralized and dispirited which results in destruction of physical

and mental coordination, so that the body is in stress, the immunity is weakened, therefore making the diseased conditions worse. After an elderly is sick, the elderly self will bears a lot of pressure, but also it brings to the family, society and medical personnel a heavy burden. If the negative sentiment of the elderly can be changed into positive sentiment, it will help to enhance their disease resistance and self-confidence. Hence it will improve the living conditions of the elder patients and enhance the quality of life. The sentiment state is a kind of psychological factor. The psychological factor is different from other factors, and its harm for the body is not directly revealed and has a hidden nature. It is invisible, and therefore people often easily overlook it. Modern medical theory and clinical practice have been converted from a pure biomedical model into a new model of 'biological - psychological - social' organic combination from the pure bio-medical model. Thus, we take measures from the psycho- logical to eliminate the patient's negative sentiment, which is very beneficial to prevention and treatment of diseases. To the end, we put forward the following measures: anxiety and frustration have a direct relationship with the hyperactivity of brain's fear center. Depression has two forms: one is reactivity, and one is internality. The reactive depression often occurs after a certain life event, such as the death of friend or relative, the fire at home, work issues, spouse's infidelity and divorce and so on, and the depressed sentiment usually does not last too long and can be recovered under correct treatment and help. The internal depression is unconsciously generated in long-term life, such as the unhappy marriage, difficult life, having chronic diseases, unsatisfactory leaders, small job title for long term, disabled child ...etc.,

MEMORY INDEX

Memory refers to the processes that are used to acquire, store, retain, and later retrieve in-formation. Human memory involves the ability to both preserve and recover in-formation we have learned or experienced. As we all know, however, this is not a flawless process. It is often understood as an informational processing system with explicit and implicit function-ing that is made up of a sensory processor, short-term (or working) memory, and long-term memory.

Memory index reflects the strength of people's memory. Cerebral arteriosclerosis, cerebral atrophy and others will lead to insufficient blood supply to the brain. The functional declina-tion of hippocampal cells in the brain is the histological reason for memory declination of the elderly. Memory is divided into two kinds: one is auditory memory that people remember by ears through listening to others' talk or read; one is visual memory that people remember by eyes through looking. An auditory dominant person remembers things they heard really well, a visual dominant person remembers things they saw really well. Memory can be divided into instantaneous memory, short-term memory and long-term memory. People do not need to preserve some memories of life in long term, sometimes we only need to remember a specific time of some things, and it's ok to forget it. But there are some things we need to maintain in our mind for a long time. If we forget some things, it will bring great difficulties and even foolish results for our study, life and work. How does memory loss occur? There are two rea-sons: one is fading; it means you forget some knowledge and do not always recall, and then the impression in the mind will gradually weaken and eventually fade away. It is like ink on a piece of paper, the ink is not always painted, so the color of ink will be light. One is interfer-ence; it means there are so many things in the mind that they are overlapped and confused; if you want to recall a problem, you cannot remember it immediately and can only remember it bit at a time after repeatedly thinking about it.

BONE DISEASE

Bone disease is a condition that damages the skeleton and makes bones weak and prone to fractures. Weak bones are not a natural part of aging. While strong bones begin in childhood, people of all ages can improve their bone health. Here are examples of several metabolic bones diseases that cause various abnormalities or deformities. Examples include osteoporosis, rickets, osteomalacia, osteogenesis im-perfecta, marble bone disease (osteopetrosis), paget disease of bone, and fibrous dysplasia.

Brittle bone disease is a lifelong genetic disorder that causes your bones to break very easily, usually without any type of injury, as from a fall. Your doctor may also call it osteogenesis imperfecta. It affects both sexes and all races equally. There is no cure for brittle bone disease, but your doctor can treat it.

TESTING TERM DESCRIPTIONS

1. Lumbar Fiber Protruding Dimension: it shows the lumbar fiber cycle or the nucleus pulposus protrudes toward one side of the body or protrudes near the side. Generally, the common case is that the left side compresses equally to the right side.

2. Adhesion Degree of Shoulder Muscle: it shows the degree of shoulder inflammatory lesions of the elderly, or the adhesion degree of shoulder muscle. Generally, the smaller the tested value is, the better it is. It proves their illness is lighter or there is no body disease.

3. Limbs Circulation Limit: it shows the limit of stiffness or activities of blood microcirculation of limbs due to a variety of external factors. Generally, four pluses mean it is most

4. serious. The less the number of plus is, the better it is; it proves that the probability of the disease factors in the body is lower.

5. Age of Ligament: this indicator is an integrated parameter obtained through the above four indicators, and the results are generally in 10% -40%. The greater value proves the degree of degenerative diseases or aging is larger, and it proves the physique and the human immunity are stronger.

Check the section of Lumbar Fiber Protruding Dimension if your client has a lower back condition where they may have a herniated disc causing the disc to shift to one side. This may show up under this reading.

If your client has a major shoulder inflammation issue, you may want to look at the Shoulder Muscle Adhesion readings. If you do some kind of therapy like osteopath, rolfing, chiropractic or massage, these readings may help confirm to your client that their condition exists and needs to be treated. Having a readout confirming what you may already know helps to solidify your client's commitment to regular treatment.

The readings of Limbs Circulation Limit and Age of Ligament section will give you more data on the state of the joints and ligament health of your client.

BONE MINERAL DENSITY ANALYSIS

REPORT OSTEOCLAST COEFFICIENT

Osteoclast consists of multinuclear giant cells that reach a diameter of 100¦Ìm, contain 2 ~ 50 nuclei and are mainly distributed in the bone surface and around bone vascular access. The osteoclasts whose number is less are combined by several single-nucleated cells, the basophilia of cytoplasm is aged following with the cells to be gradually changed to be eosinophilic. Osteoclast has a special absorption function. In absorbing some local inflammatory lesions, macrophages are also involved in the process of bone reabsorption. In the process of osteoclasts absorbing organic matters and mineral in bone matrix, the surface of matrix becomes irregular to form lacuna in a similar shape of cells, and the lacuna is called a howship. On the side toward the bone in the howship, the cells protrude a lot of hair-like protrusions which are like the longitudinal profile border and the brush border of the surface of epithelial cells. Under the electron microscope, one side close to the bone has many irregular microvilli, namely cell protrusions, being called as ruffled border. There is a circular cytoplasmic zone on the periphery of the ruffled border zone. The cytoplasmic zone contains some microfilament but lacks of other organelles, being known as clear zone where the cell membrane is smooth and is close to the bone surface. The clear zone is like a bounding wall consisting of cytoplasm and makes the surrounded area form a micro-environment. Osteoclast releases lactic acids, citric acids and others to the part. Under the acidic condition, the bone inorganic minerals are in pinocytosis from the ruffled border to form some pinocytotic vesicles or phagosomes in ruffled border matrix. In the osteoclast, the inorganic objects are degraded to be expelled into the blood stream in the form of calcium ions. The loss of inorganic objects makes collagen fibers in the bone matrix exposed. Osteoclast secretes a variety of lysosomal enzymes, especially cathepsin B and collagenolytic cathepsin. After osteoclasts leave from the bone surface, the ruffled border disappears, and the inner parts of cells are changed to enter the stationary phase. Mononuclear cells in blood or phagocytic cells in tissues cannot be transformed into osteoclasts, because all these cells only contain mature, unsplit and late mononuclear phagocytes. Only the early immature proliferating mononuclear phagocytesare the precursors of osteoclasts.

AMOUNT OF CALCIUM LOSS

In a long time, the publicity of many businessmen lets people have the impression: there is only one way to prevent and treat osteoporosis. However, after in-depth study about the pathogenesis of osteoporosis, modern medical experts find that in the pathogenesis of osteoporosis, the supplement of calcium and vitamin D as well as the impact of hormones and other non-mechanical factors are not the most important factors of the occurrence of osteo- porosis, but the muscle mass (including muscle segment mass and muscular strength) under the control of the human nervous system is one of the most important factors for determin-ing the bone strength (including bone mass and bone structure). In general, bone calcium of male after the age of 32 and female after the age of 28 begins to lose. With the increasing age, the loss rate will also be accelerated. 50% of bone calcium has been lost at 60 years old. Thus, at present, it's time to prevent fracture and prevent osteoporosis and supplement calcium. Therefore, diet nutrition is very much related to the occurrence of osteoporosis. Children and adolescents under 18 years old should take in 1200 mg of calcium each day, and adults should take in 800 mg of calcium each day. At the same time, you should take in many vitamin D to help the body more easily and more effectively absorb calcium.

DEGREE OF BONE HYPERPLASIA

It is the bone state. In the process of growth, development and functional completion of bone, some parts lose the normal shape. Bone hyperplasia has various forms and have their own characteristics because of the different parts. For instance, hyperplasia of knee joint is often referred to 'bone spur', and there is Intra-articular loose bodies and cartilage hyperplasia. Hyperplasia of spine bone mainly show the 'lip-like' change of the vertebral body, compressing the nerve, resulting in abnormal limb sense and motor abnormality.

DEGREE OF OSTEOPOROSIS

It is a phenomenon of bone reduction of the whole body. It is mainly showed that the content of bone matrix is significantly reduced, while the components of minerals (mainly containing calcium and phosphorus) in the bone are basically normal. In other words, in osteoporosis, the content of protein and other organic substances and water in the bone are decreased, and the content of calcium, phosphorus and other minerals are at the normal level. The bone matrix plays the role of support and connection between calcium, phosphorus and other minerals. Thus, if the bone matrix is reduced, the gaps among the minerals are increased, being expressed as osteoporosis. With the progress of osteo-porosis, calcium, phosphorus and other minerals in the bone will also be constantly lost and reduced, and therefore the bone matrix and minerals of the bone are decreased. Osteoporosis in old age is actually a consequence of long-term calcium deficiency.

BONE MINERAL DENSITY

This mainly reflects the strength of bone, and therefore it is the gold standard of the diag-nosis of osteoporosis, but also can predict the risk of the occurrence of fracture. Although the transformation of post-menopausal bone has a sudden-jump process, the biochemical indicators which can reflect this change and predict the risk of the occurrence of fracture in patients are very limited. Undoubtedly, it brings a lot of inconvenience for the follow up of clinical treatment and the development of research work. The researchers point out that the bone mineral density and the used biochemical indicators cannot fully reflect the effects of anti-osteoporosis treatment and predict the risk of the occurrence of fracture of patients. But there is no other more valuable test indicator, so the bone mineral density is still the most commonly used indicator for diagnosis and follow up. Determining and reflecting the bio-chemical indicators of transformation of the bone possess an important position both in the diagnosis of osteoporosis and the re-search of etiology or treatment.

In assessing older clients and particularly older females, the readings of this section are cru-cial. Amount of Calcium Loss, Osteoporosis, Bone Mineral Density and Bone Hyperplasia readings are important. You are able to see how much calcium loss has occurred in your cli-ent. If the readings are high for most of this section, you definitely want to start your client on some high absorption mineral, calcium supplements and a high mineral food diet. In addition, it would be good for them to start on a resistance exercise program as this really makes a difference in increasing bone density.

RHEUMATOID BONE DISEASE

Rheumatoid Arthritis (RA) is the most common form of autoimmune arthritis. It affects more than 1.3 million Americans. About 75% of RA patients are women. In fact, 1 – 3% of women may get rheumatoid arthritis in their lifetime. The disease most often begins between the ages of 30 and 50. However, RA can start at any age.

RA is a chronic disease that causes joint pain, stiffness, swelling and decreased movement of the joints. Small joints in the hands and feet are most commonly affected. Sometimes RA can affect your organs, such as eyes, skin or lungs.

The joint stiffness in active RA is often the worst in the morning. It may last one to two hours (or even the whole day). It generally improves with movement of the joints. Stiffness for a long time in the morning is a clue that you may have RA, as this is not common in other con-ditions. For instance, osteoarthritis most often does not cause prolonged morning stiffness

Other signs and symptoms that can occur in RA include:

• Loss of energy
• Low fevers
• Loss of appetite
• Dry eyes and mouth from a related health problem, Sjogren's syndrome
• Firm lumps, called rheumatoid nodules, which grow beneath the skin in places such as the elbow and hands
• Rheumatoid arthritis (RA) is the most common type of autoimmune arthritis. It is caused when the immune system (the body's defense system) is not working properly. RA causes pain and swelling in the wrist and small joints of the hand and feet.
• Treatments for RA can stop joint pain and swelling. Treatment also prevents joint dam-age. Early treatment will give better long term results.

•   Regular low-impact exercises, such as walking, and exercises can increase muscle strength. This will improve your overall health and lower pressure on your joints.

•   Studies show that people who receive early treatment for RA feel better sooner and more often, and are more likely to lead an active life. They also are less likely to have the type of joint damage that leads to joint replacement.

•   It is important to get the help of a rheumatologist. A rheumatologist is a doctor who treats arthritis and autoimmune disease. There are diseases that can be mistaken for RA. It is important to get the correct diagnosis without unnecessary testing. A rheumatologist will help find a treatment plan that is best for your disease.

DEGREE OF CERVICAL CALCIFICATION

It shows the size of deposit rate of cervical bone hyperplasia (increased number of cells compared to normal) No calcification means there is no hyperplasia, basic calcification means the rate of hyperplasia reaches over 30%, and calcification means the rate of hyperplasia reaches over 70%. This is not good.

As people age, the ligaments of the spine can thicken and harden , (called calcification especially in the neck cervical and lower spine area. Bones and joints may also enlarge, and bone spurs (called osteophytes) may form. Bulging or herniated discs are also common. Spondylolisthesis (the slipping of one vertebra onto another) also occurs and leads to compression)

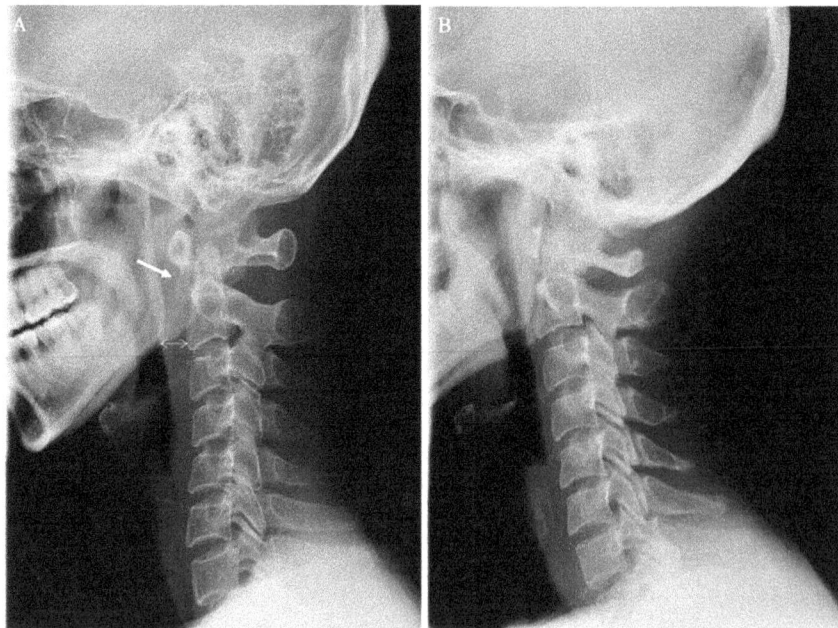

(A)Lateral radiograph of the cervical spine showing dense intervertebral disc calcification con-fined at the C5-6 (arrow). (B) Initial MRI showing round and oval shape intervertebral disc calcification at the C5-6 (arrow). (C, D) One year follow up radiograph and CT scan showing markedly decrease of the calcified disc of the C5-6 (arrow).

DEGREE OF LUMBAR CALCIFICATION

It shows the size of deposition rate of lumbar bone hyperplasia. No calcification means there is any hyperplasia, basic calcification means the rate of hyperplasia reaches over 30%, and calcification means the rate of hyperplasia reaches over 70%.

DEGREE OF HYPERPLASIA COEFFICIENT

It is the bone state. In the process of growth, development and functional completion of bone, some parts lose the normal shape. Bone hyperplasia is in various forms and has their own characteristics because of the different parts. For instance, hyperplasia of knee joint is often referred to 'bone spur', and there is Intra-articular loose bodies and cartilage hyperplasia. Hyperplasia of spine bone mainly show the 'lip-like' change of the vertebral body, compressing the nerve, resulting in abnormal limb sense and motor abnormality.

OSTEOPOROSIS COEFFICIENT

It is a phenomenon of bone reduction of the whole body. It is mainly showed that the content of bone matrix is significantly reduced, while the components of minerals (mainly containing calcium and phosphorus) in the bone are basically normal. In other words, in osteoporosis, the content of protein and other organic substances and water in the bone are decreased, and the content of calcium, phosphorus and other minerals are at the normal level. The bone matrix plays the role of support and connection between calcium, phosphorus and other minerals. Thus, if the bone matrix is reduced, the gaps among the minerals are increased, being expressed as osteoporosis. With the progress of osteo-porosis, calcium, phosphorus and other minerals in the bone will also be constantly lost and reduced, and therefore the bone matrix and minerals of the bone are decreased. Osteoporosis in old age is actually a consequence of long-term calcium deficiency. In general, bone calcium of male after the age of 32 and female after the age of 28 begins to lose. With the increasing age, the loss rate will also be accelerated. 50% of bone calcium has been lost at 60 years old. Thus, at present, it's time to prevent fracture and prevent osteoporosis and supplement calcium. Therefore, diet nutrition is very much related to the occurrence of osteoporosis. Children and adolescents under 18 years old should take in 1200 mg of calcium each day, and adults should take in 800 mg of calcium each day.

At the same time, it is need to take in many vitamins d to help the body more easily and more effectively absorb calcium.

Helping people rebuild from the inside out.

RHEUMATISM COEFFICIENT

Rheumatism is divided into the broad and the narrow. The broad rheumatism refers to a group of diseases impacting bone joints and their surrounding soft tissues, such as muscle tendon, bursae synovialis, fascia, etc. The narrow rheumatism refers to a re-current acute or chronic systemic inflammatory disease of connective tissue induced by the upper respiratory tract infection caused by Group A hemolytic streptococcus. The most obvious symptom is heart and joint lesions, significant heart valve diseases are often left to form chronic rheumatic valvular heart disease.

BONE GROWTH INDEX

BONE ALKALINE PHOSPHATASE

Bone alkaline phosphatase is secreted by the bone, it can directly reflect the activity of osteocytes, or functional status, is used as the best indicator of bone mineralization disorders to evaluate the human body.

When calcium precipitation in the bones is insufficient, the enzyme secretion increase, the secretion of calcium in bone is to reduce, so to help check for the calcium absorption.

BONE ALKALINE PHOSPHATASE

Bone alkaline phosphatase is secreted by the bone, it can directly reflect the activity of osteocytes, or functional status, is used as the best indicator of bone mineralization disorders to evaluate the human body.

When calcium precipitation in the bones is insufficient, the enzyme secretion increase, the secretion of calcium in bone is to reduce, so to help check for the calcium absorption.

OSTEOCALCIN

Value changes with ages, osteocalcin and bone changes in the different update rates. The faster the bone turnover rate, the higher the value of osteocalcin, lower in people with primary osteoporosis. For postmenopausal women, high conversion type osteo-porosis, so the osteocalcin significantly increases; for senile adult's osteoporosis has a low conversion type, thus increased osteocalcin is not obvious.

The scan can identify whether changes in osteocalcin osteoporosis is a low or high convex

STATUS OF LONG BONE HEALING

Mainly the bones of the limbs, they are like an elongated tube. They can be divided into one backbone\two ends. Body also known as the backbone of its external perimembranous bone, the central bone marrow cavity to accommodate the bone marrow.

More swollen at both ends, called epiphyseal. Epiphyseal cartilage attached to the surface of the section, the formation of the articular surface, and adjacent bone of the articular surface constitute a flexible joint movement, to complete a wide range of movement.

SHORT BONE CARTILIDGE HEALING SITUATION

These are short bones and are columnar or cuboidal bones and more groups are located in the wrist, foot, and the latter part of the spine, etc.. The short bone can withstand greater pressure, often with multiple articular surface and bone formation adjacent to the micro-joints, and often supplemented by tough ligaments, form a suitable support of flexibility of the structure that it constitutes.

EPIPHYSEAL LINE

Epiphyseal line-This is the cross-section images of the epiphyseal plate of the bone. Between the metaphysis and epiphysis of long bones have a discoid cartilage, called epiphyseal plate. In the growth, although the epiphyseal plate is in a gradual ossification, but changes itself and is less (thin), so as to ensure our long bone growth, when puberty occurs it begins to develop over time, with the sex hormone secretion, it can be understood as the epiphysis. After the gradual ossification of the bone, it does not continue to grow, all ossification is finished, and no longer is there space and material for growth.

I would only use this section if your client has a bone growth issue. If your client is a teenager or child dealing with bone healing issues or a growth condition, look at these readings. Refer to the definition section as well.

BLOOD SUGAR ANALYSIS

COEFFCIENT OF INSULIN SECRETION

Insulin is a kind of protein hormone. Pancreatic β-cells are secreted into insulin in the body. Beside the duodenum of the body, there is a long-shaped organ called as pancreas. Many cell masses are scattered in the pancreas, and the cell mass is called as pancreatic islet. There are about 100 to 200 million pancreatic islets in the pancreas. Islet cells are divided into the following categories in accordance with their functions for secreting hormones: (1) B-cell (β cells), accounting for about 60% to 80% of islet cells, and secreting insulin which can lower blood sugar. (2) A cell (α cells), accounting for about 24% to 40% of islet cells, and secreting glucagon which has the contrary role of insulin and can increase blood sugar. (3) D cell, accounting for about 6% to 15% of the total number of islet cells, and secreting growth hormone-inhibiting hormone. Due to viral infection, autoimmune, genetic and other disease factors, the pathophysiology of diabetes patients is mainly caused by relative or absolute lack

Of insulin activity and relative or absolute excess glucagon activity, namely B and A cell bilateral hormone dysfunction. Insulin-dependent diabetes in which insulin-secreting cells are in severe damage or complete absence, such as lower endogenous insulin secretion, needs exogenous insulin therapy. In non-insulin-dependent diabetes, insulin secretion disorder is lighter, the concentration of basal insulin is normal or is elevated, insulin secretion is generally lower than that of persons of the corresponding weight after glucose stimulation, namely the relative lack of insulin. The insulin secretion function has an important reference value in diabetes diagnosis, classification, treatment, prognosis and predication for high-risk groups whether they will have diabetes in future. Both clinicians and researchers attach importance to its assessment. The level of insulin secretion is impacted by both insulin resistance and β cell function.

BLOOD SUGAR COEFFICIENT
Blood sugar refers to the glucose in blood. Other types of sugar, such as sugar, di-saccharide and polysaccharides can be called as glucose after they are converted into glucose to enter into blood. The blood glucose concentration of the healthy human body is also in a stable and balanced state. Once the balance is destroyed, such as abnormally increased glucose, diabetes will appear.

URINE SUGAR COEFFICIENT
Urine sugar refers to the sugar in urine, mainly referring to the glucose in urine. The healthy human body's urine sugar is little, it cannot be measured by the general method, so the healthy human body's urine sugar is negative or there is no sugar in urine. In the healthy human body, only when blood sugar is over 160 ~ 180mg/dl, more sugar can be excreted from the urine to form urine sugar. Therefore, the blood sugar level determines the presence or absence of urine sugar.

I look at this section's readings if the client is a diabetic or has all the characteristics of a borderline diabetic. You want to see that sugar levels and insulin levels are in the normal range.

TRACE ELEMENTS
Calcium(Ca):
Calcium is a metallic element, being silver-white crystal and being easy for chemical combination. For instance, animal bones, clam shells and eggshells contain calcium carbohydrate, calcium phosphate, etc. Calcium is one of constant elements of the body and it accounts for fifth place of the trace elements in the body.
The role of calcium in the body:
1. It composes the human skeleton and supports the body, being the fulcrum of muscle flexing.

2. In the soft tissue of blood cells, it plays important roles, such as heart rate maintenance, nerve conduction, muscle contraction, blood coagulation and cell adhesion. Unfortunately, although it is very important, it can be synthesized by the body only by external intake.

Iron(Fe):
Iron accounts for fifth place of the trace elements in the body. It is the necessary matter for constituting hemoglobin, cell chromatin and tissue enzyme and has the oxygen carrier function. Iron deficiency can cause anemia, lower oxygen carrier function and cause tissue hypoxia which cause diseases. A healthy adult's body contains 3-5g of iron, and a healthy baby's body contains 500mg.

Zinc(Zn):
Zinc as an important trace element in the human body's composition and it's an activator composing hundreds of kinds of enzymes in the body. Its main function: it catalyzes human biochemical reactions, activates various enzyme proteins and is involved in protein synthesis to promote active metabolism.

Zinc deficiency can cause:
1. Dull sense of taste and blocking of the taste buds of the tongue
2. Partial eclipse and pica, such as eating cinders, mud, nails, plaster, etc.
3. Dwarfism
4. It is difficult to heal wounds.
5. Hypoplasia of secondary sexual characteristic (when secondary sexual characteristics fail to develop during puberty)
6. Women's menstrual cramps, or amenorrhea
7. It affects the sperm motility to cause sterility.

Selenium(Se):
Selenium is one of the necessary trace elements of the human body. Selenium is a carrier of calcium, and calcium cannot be attached on the bone if there is no selenium. Selenium can help to activate antioxidant enzymes, such as glutathione peroxidase, which can neutralize potentially harmful free radicals. Selenium is the necessity for maintenance of muscle (including heart) health. Selenium also has a certain effect in maintaining eyesight, skin and hair health.

Human selenium deficiency can have a variety of expressive modes, and the common expressive modes include: myalgia, myositis, myocardial fatty change, Keshan disease, hemolytic anemia, bone changes (Kashin-Beck disease), etc. Leukocyte bactericidal capacity and cell-mediated immunity is reduced therefore infection can occur.

Phosphorus(P):
Almost all of the foods contain phosphorus. Plenty of phosphorus can be obtained in diet. A supplement is not needed. The excessive intake of phosphorus will destroy the balance of minerals and cause calcium deficiency. Especially in people over the age of 40, the kidneys can no longer help to excrete excess phosphorus, which will lead to calcium deficiency. Therefore, the meat intake should be reduced, and more milk and vegetables should be taken.
Too much phosphorus in the blood will reduce the concentration of calcium, which will cause hypocalcemia, leading to enhanced neural excitability, tetany (intermittent muscular spasms) and convulsion. The manifestations are: 1. Brittle and Fragile bones; 2. Tooth decay; 3. Various symptoms resulting from calcium deficiency become increasingly evident; 4. Nervous breakdown; 5. The unbalance of other minerals.

Potassium(K):
Potassium is an essential macronutrient in human. The content of potassium in an adult body is about 150 g. Potassium is stored mainly in the body cells. It is an essential nutrient in human body and an important electrolyte for the organism. The main function of it is maintaining and regulating volume and osmotic pressure of the intracellular fluid, maintaining acid base balance of humor (fluid or semi-fluid substance) and the con-duction of nerve actions. Potassium plays very important roles on the metabolism and the maintenance of the structure and function of human cells. It can enhance the excitability of human nerve and muscle, reducing myocardial excitability, so it can maintain the normal function of nerves and muscles, especially the normal movement of the heart.
Normally the concentration of serum potassium is 3.5 to 5.5 mmol / l, and the symptom of the concentration of potassium lower than 3.5 mmol / l is called hypokalemia. The most outstanding manifestation of hypokalemia is limb numbness with different levels of neuro muscular relaxation and paralysis, especially in the crura (which is one of two tendinous structures that extends below the diaphragm to the vertebral column. There is a right crus and a left crus, which together form a tether for muscular contraction). This is called potassium-deficiency-caused flaccid paralysis. It usually starts from the lower extremities, especially from the quadriceps, with the symptoms of weak standing ability, weakness or difficulty ascending. Then with the aggravation of the potassium deficiency, muscle weakness can be more seri- ous: the loss of muscle strength of trunk and upper limbs; becoming serious gradually until it effects the respiratory muscles, or even leads to respiratory failure, or accompanied by severe dysfunction of the cardiovascular system, such as chest tightness, palpitation, and even res- piratory muscle paralysis, difficulty breathing and severe arrhythmia.

Magnesium(Mg):

In human cells, magnesium is the second most important cation (with potassium first). The content of magnesium is inferior to that of potassium. Magnesium has many special physiological functions: it can activate a variety of enzymes in the body, inhibit abnormal excitation of nerve system, maintain the stability of the structure of nuclear acids, and participate in protein synthesis, muscle contraction and body temperature regulation. Magnesium affects the [channel] for the intra and extra cellular mobility of potassium, sodium and calcium, and maintains the membrane potential.

The clinical manifestations of magnesium deficiency are: emotional disturbance, ex-citation, tetany, hyperreflexia, etc. Normally oral intake of overdose of magnesium will not lead to magnesium toxicity due to the regulation of the kidney. But in circumstance of renal insufficiency, a large number of oral magnesium can cause magnesium toxicity, manifested as abdominal pain, diarrhea, vomiting, polydipsia, fatigue, weakness, and difficulty in breathing, cyanosis, mydriasis etc. in serious situation.

Copper(Cu):

The manifestations of copper deficiency are hypochromic small-cell anemia, stunted growth, bone lesions such as arthritis, proliferation and bone fractures, ulcer, hepatosplenomegaly, cardiovascular damage, coronary heart disease, brain barrier, vitiligo, and female infertility. If the copper intake exceeds 100 times more than the requirement for the human body it will cause hemolytic anemia and necrotizing hepatitis. The poisoning symptoms of copper are salivation, nausea and vomiting, hematemesis, bellyache and diarrhea, acute gastroenteritis, hemolysis, hematuria, melena, red protein in the urinary, lysosomal membrane rupture, jaundice, arrhythmia, liver tissue necrosis, renal failure, uremia and shock. Excessive copper can not only cause schizophrenia, epilepsy and rheumatoid arthritis, but also related to tumors including esophageal cancer, gastric cancer, liver cancer and lung cancer. The toxicosis of overdose of copper can be treated by gastric lavage with dimercaptopropanol and potassium ferrocyanide or sodium thiosulfate.

Cobalt(Co):

Cobalt is the essential element of the human body. It exists in a state of ion. Cobalt is a component of vitamin B12, related to hematopoietic function. The daily intake of cobalt in human body is about 5 - 45 mg. Intake of overdose of cobalt will induce pneumonia, and lead to myocardial damage, thyroid damage and erythrocytosis, etc. Co-60¦Ã-ray has certain effects on the treatment of human cancer.

Manganese(Mn):

The Mn deficiency in human body will affect the growth and development. Mn deficiency in pregnant women causes baby Mn deficiency, which will lead to ataxia in newborns; Mn deficiency in children and adolescents may impair growth and lead to bone deformities; Mn deficiency in adults may cause reproductive dysfunction. Although the sea is very rich in manganese, and manganese plays an important role in human body, the body's requirement for manganese is very tiny. The manganese requirement in diet of ordinary people is 4-9 mg per day, about half of which is absorbed by intestine.

Manganese is also involved in hematopoiesis. The mechanism of manganese in hematopoiesis is by improving the body utilization of copper to promote the absorption and utilization of iron and maturation and release of red blood cells.

Iodine(I):

Iodine is an essential micronutrient. The content of iodine in adults is about 20 to 50 mg, 70% to 80% of which concentrates in the thyroid near the throat, the rest presenting in muscle and other tissues. Iodine is the essential material for the synthesis of thyroid hormone, the deficiency of which can lead to hypothyroidism, causing mental and physical developmental dis- abilities. deficiency in children will affect their growth and development; deficiency in pregnant women will not only result in goiter in herself but also affect fetal development, leading to slow growth, dwarfism, deafness, mental retardation, and even dementia in children after birth, which is called [cretinism]; goiter in adults can reduce the body's energy metabolism, causing myxedema, heart rate reduction, decreased sexual function, facial swelling and slow speech.

The daily supply of iodine for adults is about 100 to 200 mg, and that for children aged 1 to 10 is 60 ~110 mg. Excessive iodine intake may cause iodine goiter, so the iodine intake is not the much, the better. Iodine-rich food is seafood, such as kelp, seaweed, sea fish and sea salt. The iodine concentration of seaweed is thousands times higher than that of seawater. Iodine also exists in the soil of most areas. So the daily requirement for iodine can be obtained in vegetables and water as well.

Nickel(Ni):

Nickel is an essential element of life, mainly supplied by vegetable, cereal and seaweed, etc. Nickel is widely distributed in nature, but its content in the human body is extremely low. Normally, the adult body contains about 10mg of nickel, and the daily requirement for nickel is 0.3mg. Lack of nickel can cause diabetes mellitus, anemia, cirrhosis, uremia, renal failure and metabolic dysfunction of liver lipid and phospholipids, etc. Animal experiments showed that lack of nickel will cause slow growth, rising mortality rate of the organism, decrease of hematocrit, hemoglobin and iron content, reduce the bone calcium content and the zinc content in liver, hair, muscles and bones, and brain. Nickel deficiency is one of the causes of infertility.

Fluorine(F):

Fluorine is a nonmetallic element. The main toxic symptoms caused by excessive fluoride in human body are: yellow teeth, black teeth, X-or O-shaped legs, crookback or arm with dysfunction in stretching, dental fluorosis in mild sufferers, skeletal fluorosis in severe sufferers who might even lost the abilities of working and living. One suffering from fluorosis once will never be cured, and medications can only slow the aggravation of the disease. Endemic fluorosis is an endemic seriously endangering the health of people, which is a biogeochemical disease, divided into water-drinking type, coal-burning type and tea-drinking type.

Molybdenum(Mo):

Molybdenum is one of the essential micronutrients. The total molybdenum content in adult body is about 9 mg, distributed in various tissues and fluids of the body, in which liver and kidney contains the highest content of molybdenum, Molybdenum requirements of the body is very small, and molybdenum exists in a variety of foods. Molyb-denum functions as the prosthetic group of enzymes, catalytically oxidating the cor-responding substrate. Molybdenum deficiency will not occur under normal conditions, but may occur in long-term total parenteral nutrition patients (where nutrition is ad-ministered in a manner other than through digestive tract, as by intravenous or in-tramuscular injection). Lack of molybdenum in animals can cause weight loss, reduced fertility, and shortened life expectancy.

Vanadium(V):

Vanadium is one of the essential micronutrients, playing important roles on the maintenance of body growth and development, acceleration on the growth of bones and teeth, and promotion on hematopoiesis and the increase of body immunity. The proper amount of vanadium can also lower blood sugar, blood pressure and lipids, increasing myocardial contractility and preventing heart disease. At present what researchers are most concerned with is its hypogly-cemic function. Insulin is the only hormone to reduce blood glucose in human body. Vanadi-um can not only play a role as insulin, but also protect the islet cells, thus reducing the body blood sugar.

Daily diet provides about 15 mg of vanadium, which can meet the body's requirements, and supplement of vanadium is not needed. But people lacking vanadium or patients with diabetes, high cholesterol and hypertension should pay attention to take vanadium in foods. Cereal products, meat, chicken, duck, fish, cucumber, shellfish, mushrooms and parsley contain plenty of vanadium. But inorganic vanadium salt has unsatisfied fat-solubility, bad absorption, and great toxicity, which will affect people's health.

Tin(Sn):

Tin is an essential micronutrient of human lives, and one of the earliest elements human found as well. Recent scientific research shows that: tin can improve the metabolism of protein and nucleic acid, conducive to growth and development. Lack of tin leads to slow development of the body, especially for children. Tin deficiency will affect the normal development, and in severe cases can cause dwarfism.

Silicon(Si):

Silicon is an essential mineral in the human body and a micronutrient as well. Silicon maintains flexibility and elasticity of our bodies, making us possess soft skin and hard bone. Silicone can promote child growth and development, and also plays an irreplaceable role in the prevention of aging. Besides, silicon can promote the increase of collagen, resulting in some cosmetic effects. Lack of silicon will lead to dry skin, wrinkling and susceptibleness to fractures. With the growth of age, silicon content in various tissues gradually decreased. Thus, the reduction degree of silicon content can be used as an indicator for aging to remind the elderly to enhance healthcare and anti-aging.

The harm of silicon to human body is made by the lack of silicon or excessive silicon. Silicon shortage may cause osteoporosis and fragile nails etc. But excessive silicon is also very harmful. For example the long-term inhalation of dioxide silicon dust will easily cause excessive silicon, leading to silicosis. Excessive silicon in body may result in focal glomerulonephritis.

Strontium(Sr):

Strontium is an essential micronutrient, which can promote the growth and development of the bone. In long-term people have been focus only on the relativity between bone development and VD and calcium, but neglected the importance of strontium. The latest research data shows that: the lack of strontium human body will lead to metabolic disorders, and will cause physical weakness, sweating and skeletal growth retardation, even resulting in serious consequences such as osteoporosis.

The research concludes that: children's insufficient intake of coarse grains and vegetables matching with food, blindly supplied with calcium supplements are the main causes of children strontium deficiency. To avoid the lack of strontium, children should pay attention to the thickness of grain and the kinds of meat and vegetables, and take the calcium supplements with dairy products and animal bones under the guidance of a doctor or health practitioner.

Boron(B):

Boron commonly exists in fruits and vegetables, which is one of the micronutrients to maintain the health of the bone and metabolism of calcium, phosphorus and magnesium. The lack of boron will increase the lack of vitamin C; on the other hand, boron also helps to im- prove the secretion of testosterone, strengthen the muscles, which is an essential nutrient for athletes. Boron also improves the brain function and enhances the reaction capacity. Although most people do not lack boron, it is necessary for the elderly to take proper amount of boron.

It is important that you check this section because many people are low in calcium, iron, zinc and selenium. If the readings are low, you may want to advise your clients on good natural supplements and a high mineral diet of more raw foods, juices, etc.

VITAMIN ANALYSIS

Vitamin A:
Vitamin A is related to growth and reproduction, and is an indispensable material of epithelial cells. The lack of vitamin A will cause cortex keratosis, rough skin, night blindness and dry eye.

Vitamin B1:
Vitamin B1 is in charge of carbohydrate metabolism. The lack of vitamin B1 will make the substance not metabolized accumulate in the tissues to result in poisoning, athlete's foot, feet numbness, edema and weakened functions of muscle, skin or heart.

Vitamin B2:
Vitamin B2 is in charge of fat and protein metabolism and detoxification in the liver. The lack of vitamin B2 will cause decreased growth and skin type and mouth type digestive disturbances.

Vitamin B3:
Vitamin B3 is also known as nicotinic acid and nicotinamide. It can be dissolved in water and can make use of tryptophan for synthesis in the human body, and it is an essential substance of synthetic hormones. Vitamin B3 can promote blood circulation, lower blood pressure, lower cholesterol and triglycerides, reduce gastrointestinal disorder and alleviate the symptoms of Meniere's syndrome and so on. Vitamin B3 has effects for seborrheic dermatitis and eczema and the functions for whitening and activating the skin cells. Vitamin B3 exists in animal livers, kidneys, lean meat, eggs, wheat germ, whole wheat products, peanuts, figs, etc.

Vitamin B6:

Vitamin B6 is related to amino acid metabolism. It can lead to disappearance of neurological irritability and have a certain role for the formation of immune substances and the prevention of arterioschlerosis. The lack of vitamin B6 will cause anemia, frostbite and other skin disorders. In addition, it can inhibit tryptophan to convert into xanthurenic acid damaging the pancreas, thereby protecting the pancreas.

Vitamin B12:

Vitamin B12 has the function for stimulating the hematopoietic function of bone marrow.
Vitamin C (Ascorbic acid):
Vitamin C is colorless crystal, can be dissolved in water and alcohol, and can be easily destroyed. Its main functions: it can enhance the body immunity and protect capillaries, prevent scurvy and promote wound healing. Vitamin C can increase the use of iron, its chemical and biological process is that it reduces ferric iron in the diet to ferrous iron to promote the absorption of iron and to store iron in ferritin in the liver and bones. Practice shows that the supplementation of iron as well as adding VC can increase the iron absorption rate by 22%, it basically reaches the normal absorption rate of hemoglobin.

Vitamin D3:

Its main physiological function is to promote intestinal calcium absorption, induce bone calcium-phosphorus attaching and prevent rickets.

Vitamin E:

Its basic function is to protect the integrity of the internal structure of cells, and it can inhibit the oxidation of lipid in cells and on cell membranes and protect cells against damage of free radical. It also has the functions of anti-oxidation, anti-aging and beautifying.

Vitamin K:

Vitamin K is an important vitamin for promoting normal blood coagulation and bone growth. Vitamin K is the essential substance in the synthesis of four kinds of blood clotting proteins (prothrombin, factor VII, anti-hemophilia factor and stuart factor) in the liver. The human body has little vitamin K, but it can maintain normal function of blood coagulation, reduce heavy bleeding in the physiological period, and prevent internal bleeding and hemorrhoids. The person with frequent nosebleed should take in more vitamin K from the natural foods.

Vitamin A:

Vitamin A is related to growth and reproduction, and is an indispensable material of epithelial cells. The lack of vitamin A will cause cortex keratosis, rough skin, night blindness and dry eye.

Vitamin B1:
Vitamin B1 is in charge of carbohydrate metabolism. The lack of vitamin B1 will make the substance not metabolized, accumulate in the tissues to result in poisoning, athlete's foot, feet numbness, edema and weakened functions of muscle, skin or heart.

Vitamin B2:
Vitamin B2 is in charge of fat and protein metabolism and detoxification in the liver. The lack of vitamin B2 will cause decreased growth and skin type and mouth type digestive disturbances.

Vitamin B3:
Vitamin B3 is also known as nicotinic acid and nicotinamide. It can be dissolved in water and can make use of tryptophan for synthesis in the human body, and it is an essential substance of synthetic hormones. Vitamin B3 can promote blood circulation, lower blood pressure, lower cholesterol and triglycerides, reduce gastrointestinal disorder and alleviate the symptoms of Meniere's syndrome and so on. Vitamin B3 deficiency can cause seborrheic dermatitis and eczema. It also functions in whitening and activating the skin cells. Vitamin B3 exists in animal livers, kidneys, lean meat, eggs, wheat germ, whole wheat products, peanuts, figs, etc.

Vitamin B6:
Vitamin B6 is related to amino acid metabolism. It can lead to disappearance of neurological irritability and have a certain role for the formation of immune substances and the prevention of arterioschlerosis. The lack of vitamin B6 will cause anemia, frostbite and other skin disorders. In addition, it can inhibit tryptophan to convert into xanthurenic acid damaging the pancreas, thereby protecting the pancreas.

Vitamin B12:
Vitamin B12 has the function for stimulating the hematopoietic function of bone marrow.
Vitamin C (Ascorbic acid):
Vitamin C is colorless crystal, can be dissolved in water and alcohol, and can be easily destroyed. Its main functions: it can enhance the body's immunity and protect capillaries, pre- vent scurvy and promote wound healing. Vitamin C can increase the use of iron, its chemical and biological process is that it reduces ferric iron in the diet to ferrous iron to promote the absorption of iron and to store iron as ferritin in the liver and bones. Practice shows that the supplementation of iron as well as adding Vitamin C can increase the iron absorption rate by

22%, it basically reaches the normal absorption rate of hemoglobin.

Vitamin D3:

Its main physiological function is to promote intestinal calcium absorption, induce bone calcium-phosphorus, attacking and preventing rickets.

Vitamin E:

Its basic function is to protect the integrity of the internal structure of cells, and it can inhibit the oxidation of lipid in cells and on cell membranes and protect cells against damage of free radical. It also has the functions of anti-oxidation, anti-aging and beautifying.

Vitamin K:

Vitamin K is an important vitamin for promoting normal blood coagulation and bone growth. Vitamin K is the essential substance in the synthesis of four kinds of blood clotting proteins (prothrombin, factor VII, anti-hemophilia factor and stuart factor) in the liver. The human body has little vitamin K, but it can maintain normal function of blood coagulation, reduce heavy bleeding in the physiological period, and prevent internal bleeding and hemorrhoids. The person with frequent nosebleed should take in more vitamin K from the natural foods.

It is essential you check this section since it is directly related to proper nutrition. If a client has low readings in any of the B vitamins or in vitamin C, I suggest you have them supplement with a 50 mg vitamin B complex and vitamin C powder to bring levels up. These two vitamins are water soluble and usually lost from the body within 48 hours. It's important to replace the vitamins. Also, if any of the other vitamins are low, suggest to your client to take that extra vitamin supplement. For more detailed information of each vitamin, refer to the definition section of Vitamins in thisbook.

AMINO ACID ANALYSIS

Lysine:

Lysine enhances the development of the brain. It is the composition of liver and gallbladder, which enhances the metabolism of the fats, regulates the pineal gland, lactiferous glands, corpus luteum and ovary, and prevent the degradation of the cell.

Lysine is the basic essential amino acid. Due to the low content in the cereal and the destruction during the food processing lysine is deficient, so it is called the first limiting amino acid. Symptoms for lack of lysine include fatigue, weakness, nausea, vomiting, dizziness, loss of appetite, growth retardation and anemia. Nutritious supplements can be taken in the advice of the medical professionals. The recommended intake for lysine is 10mg/pound for children,

3000-9000mg for adults. Lysine is the key material helpful to the absorption and utilization of other nourishment. Only when the body is supplied with sufficient lysine, the protein absorption and utilization of food can be enhanced, the nutrition can be balanced, and growth and development can be promoted.

Lysine may adjust the balance of the human body metabolism. Lysine provides structural components for the synthesis of carnitine, which will lead to the synthesis of fatty acids in cells. Adding a small amount of lysine in foods will stimulate the secretion of pepsin and acid and improve the gastric secretion, which can enhance appetite and promote the growth and development of the infants. Lysine also increases absorption and accumulation of calcium in the body, accelerate bone growth. Lack of lysine may cause low gastric secretion, which will lead to anorexia and nutritional anemia, resulting in central nervous system disruption and dysplasia.

Tryptophan:

It promotes the production of gastric and pancreatic juice. Tryptophan can be converted to an important neurotransmitter in human brain ----5 - hydroxy tryptamine, which can act as norepinephrine and epinephrine and can improve the sleep duration. When the content of 5 - ht decreases in the brain of an animal, the abnormal behavior, insanity hallucinations and insomnia will occur. In addition, 5 - ht has a strong effect of vasoconstriction. It may exist in many tissues, including platelets and intestinal mucosa cells. The injured organism will stanch bleeding by the release of 5 - ht. Tryptophan is often used as anti-nausea agent, anticonvulsant, gastric secretion regulator, gastric mucosal protection agent and strong anti-coma agent.

Phenylalanine:

It participates in eliminating the loss of the function of kidney and bladder. Phenylalanine is one of the essential amino acids for human body. Ingested through food intake, some of the phenylalanine are used for protein synthesis, and the rest are converted into tyrosine in reaction with liver tyrosine hydroxylase, and then converted into other bio-logically active substances.

Methionine:

It is the constituent of hemoglobin, tissue and serum and it supports the function of the spleen, pancreas and lymph.

Methionine is a sulfur-containing essential amino acid, closely related to the in-vivo metabolism of a variety of sulfur compounds. The lack of methionine will cause loss of appetite, growth-slowing or stagnation of weight-gaining, enlarged kidney and liver iron accumulation. Then it can lead to liver necrosis or fibrosis.

Methionine can also be methylate which is toxic or a drug with its methyl to perform the function of detoxification. Thus, methionine can be used in the prevention and treatment of liver diseases such as chronic or acute hepatitis and cirrhosis, etc, and in the alleviation of the toxicity of harmful substances such as arsenic, chloroform, carbohydrate tetrachloride, benzene, pyridine and quinoline and so on.

Threonine:

This has the function of converting some of the amino acids to gain the balance of amino acids in the body. Threonine has a hydroxyl in its structure, which retains water in human skin. Combining with the oligosaccharide chain, it plays an important role in protecting the cell membrane, and promotes in-vivo phospholipid synthesis and fatty acid oxidation. Its preparation has the medicinal function of enhancing human body development and resisting fatty liver, being a composition of the composite amino acid infusion. Meanwhile, threonine is the raw material to produce streptozotocina, an antibiotic with high efficiency and low allergenic- ity.

Isoleucine:

It participates in the regulation and metabolism of thymus, spleen and pituitary gland. Valine, leucine and isoleucine are branched-chain amino acids, and essential amino acids as well. Isoleucine can be used in the treatments of neurological disorders, loss of appetite and anemia, has an important role in muscle protein metabolism.

You want to look at the amino acid levels to make sure they are in the normal range. The 9 essential amino acids are found in protein foods. Each has an important function. For example, the amino acid, Valine, is crucial in preventing muscle break down during exercise or physical activity. In many cases, female clients are low in some of the amino acids because they do not eat enough protein. This is where I recommend protein whey isolate supplements to people to get the extra protein they need.

COENZYME ANALYSIS

Nicotinamide:

Nicotinamide is an essential coenzyme in vivo, plays a role in the biological oxidation of hydrogen transfer, can activate a variety of enzyme systems, to promote nucleic acid, protein, polysaccharide synthesis and metabolism, increasing regulation and control of material transport and improve metabolism.

Biotin:

It is the necessary material of synthesis of vitamin C, is essential to normal metabolism of fat and protein substances. It is necessary for the body's natural growth and to maintain normal body function as water-soluble vitamins; It is an essential fat and protein metabolism of the material, also to maintain normal growth, development and health of the necessary nutri-ents.

Pantothenic acid:

It participates in the manufacture of energy in the body, and can control fat metabolism. It is necessary for brain and nerve nutrient. Helps the body anti-stress hormones (steroids) se-cre-tion. To maintain healthy skin and hair.

Folic acid:

Folic acid is the necessary material of the body's use of sugars and amino acids, it is the necessary material of the body cell growth and reproduction. Lack of folic acid can cause giant cell anemia and leukopenia to the human body, also lead to physical weakness, irritability, loss of appetite, and psychiatric symptoms.

Coenzyme Q10:

Coenzyme Q10 is a fat-soluble antioxidant, coenzyme Q10 is indispensable to human life, one of the important elements that can activate the body's cells and energy nutrients, improve immunity, enhance anti-oxidation, anti-aging and enhance the vitality of the human body, etc. function. The total body content of coenzyme Q10 is only 500-1500mg and with the elderly it is less. The organs of the human contain coenzyme Q10 at its peak at age 20 and then it starts to decrease.

Glutathione:

Glutathione is composed of three amino acid peptides, exists in almost every cell of the body. Normal glutathione helps the body maintain a normal immune system function. A major physiological role of glutathione is its important antioxidant. It can rid the body of free radicals, clean; purify the human body, environmental pollution, thus enhancing people's health. Check this section to see which nutrients your client may be low in. If they are low in any of the enzyme or antioxidant readings, you may want to direct them to the proper supplement.

ENDOCRINE SYSTEM ANALYSIS

Thyroid secretion index:

Thyroid is an important organ of the endocrine system, there is a clear distinction between Thyroid and other systems in the body (such as respiratory, etc), but it works closely with the nervous system, they interact with each other, known as the two major biological information systems, without their close cooperation, the body's internal environment cannot maintain relative stability. The endocrine glands are stimulated appropriately by nerve , can make some of these endocrine cells release chemicals efficiently, the chemical was sent to the corresponding organ by the blood circulation to play regulating functions, these highly

efficient chemical messengers are called hormones. Thyroid is the largest endocrine gland in the human endocrine system, it can secret thyroid hormones after its stimulated by nerves, and these hormones will have a physiological effect after being sent to the corresponding organ in the human body.

Parathyroid hormone secretion index:
PTH's main function is to affect the metabolism of calcium and phosphorus, mobilizing calcium from the bones to increase calcium concentration in blood, while also acting on the intestine and renal tubules to increase the absorption of calcium, so as to maintain the stability of calcium. If the parathyroid secretion is low, calcium concentration is decreased, then tetany can occur; if hyperthyroidism occurs, bones are prone to fractures. Parathyroid dysfunction may cause disorders of blood calcium and phosphorus ratio.

Adrenal glands Index:
Adrenal medulla is part of the internal, secretion of adrenaline and noradrenaline. The increased release of stress hormones, can help increase blood pressure, heart rate, elevated blood glucose, mobilize the reserve substances in the body, to prepare for struggling with the external environment. Therefore, adrenal glands are a very important in the body. All its activities are subject to the nerve center of the pituitary. For example, aldosterone secretion is regulated by the kidney's hormone renin, secretion of cortisol and androgen are regulated by ACTH of the pituitary. Epinephrine and norepinephrine are regulated by the sympathetic nervous system.

Pituitary secretion index:
Pituitary glands is the most important human gland, it has two parts: sub-frontal and posterior lobe. It secretes hormones, such as growth hormone, thyroid stimulating hormone, adrenocorticotropic hormone, gonadotropin, oxytocin, prolactin, black cell stimulating hormone, etc., can also store the antidiuretic hormone of hypothalamus secretion. These hormones play an important role on metabolism, growth, development and reproduction, etc.

Pineal Gland:
Its cells are dominated by sympathetic postganglionic fibers which form cervical ganglion. Within the pineal gland, serotonin is acetylated and then methylated to yield melatonin. Synthesis and secretion of melatonin is dramatically affected by light exposure to the eyes.

... Note that blood levels of melatonin are essentially undetectable during daytime, but rise sharply during the dark. Sympathetic stimulation may promote the synthesis and secretion of pineal melatonin. Secretion of the pineal gland is closely related to light, pineal gland will become small in the presence of light, inhibit the secretion of pineal cells and when it is dark the secretion of the pineal occurs. Since melatonin secretion and synthesis are regulated by light and darkness, so it appears secretion occurs with the circadian rhythm. In human plasma, its secretion is lowest at noon and highest at midnight. In addition, its cyclical secretion is closely related to the sexual cycle of animals and humans, as well as to the menstrual cycle of women. Pineal gland will release time signal to the central nervous system through the melatonin secretion cycle, thus affecting the body's biological effects of time, such as sleep and awakening, especially the cyclical activity of hypothalamus-pituitary-gonadal.

Thymus gland secretion index:

Thymus is a lymphoid organ with endocrine function . Thymus develops and becomes larger in the neonatal and early childhood, after sexually maturity, it will gradually shrink. Thymus is divided into left and right lobe, asymmetric, adult thymus is about 25 to 40 grams, color gray red, and soft, mainly located in the anterior mediastinum. Thymus is hematopoietic organ. In the embryonic phase and in adulthood it can produce lymphocytes, plasma cells, and myeloid cells. Thymus reticular epithelial cells secrete thymosin. It can promote the producing and maturing of T cells with immune function and it also can inhibit the synthesis and release of acetylcholine and its motor nerve terminals. When there is thymoma, thymosin will increase, this could lead to the my-asthenia gravis because of the emergence of neuromuscular disorder.

Gland secretion index:

Mainly refers to the male gonad testis and ovaries in women.

Testis secrete male hormone testosterone (testosterone), its main function is to promote the development of gonad and its subsidiary structures and the appearance of sexual characteristics, but also to promote protein synthesis.

Ovarian secrete follicle stimulating hormone, progesterone, relaxin and male hormones. Its functions are:

(1) To stimulate endometrial proliferation, to promote thickening of the uterus, enlarge breast and the emergence of female sexual characteristics and so on.
(2) To promote proliferation of uterine epithelium and uterine gland and maintain the body's water, sodium, calcium levels, and lower blood sugar, elevate body temperature.
(3) To promote the laxity of cervix and the pubic symphysis ligaments to help in childbirth.
(4) To enable women to have masculine sexual characteristics, etc.

Go to this section to see which hormone levels are low or high for your client. Refer back to the earlier section in the book on what each hormone does in the body. This may confirm why your client has some of the health issues they are experiencing. You may be able to help with some supplements and a change in diet to increase or decrease that hormone so they can reach a higher level of health and possibly decrease their negative health symptoms.

IMMUNE SYSTEM ANALYSIS

Lymph node Index:

Lymph node is the unique organ of mammals. Normal human's superficial lymph nodes is very small, smooth, so no adhesion occurs with surrounding tissue , less than 0.5 cm in diameter .

The lymph nodes are major organs that perform many functions within the lymphatic system. Primarily, they remove debris and pathogens from lymph or tissue fluid. Some people describe the lymph nodes as lymph filters because of this primary function. The organs contain many cells that can internalize and kill pathogens that pass through. Additionally, the lymph nodes act as the site for adaptive immune responses involving special types of white blood cells.

When the bacteria enter into your body from the site of injury, the lymphocytes will produce lymphokines and antibodies to kill the bacteria effectively. The result is lymphocytes hyperplasia and histiocytosis of the cellular response to lymph nodes within the lymph node, as lymph nodes become reactive resulting in hyperplasia. Viruses, certain chemicals, toxic products of metabolism, degeneration of tissue components and foreign material can cause
lymph node reactive hyperplasia. Therefore, the enlarged lymph nodes are the body's beacon, a warning device

Tonsil immune Index:

Tonsil is the largest lymphoid tissue in pharyngeal. In childhood, it is an active immune organ, containing all developmental stages of the cell, such as T cells, B cells, and phagocytic cells. It therefore has a role in humoral immunity, resulting in a variety of immune globulin, also have some role in cellular immunity. Tonsil IgA immunoglobulins produced a strong immune system, they inhibit bacterial adhesion to respiratory mucosa, and inhibit bacterial growth and spread of the virus, therefore they have a very important function in neutralization and inhibition.

Bone marrow Index:

Human hematopoietic bone marrow is located within the body's bones. There are Two types of adult bone marrow: red marrow and yellow marrow. Red bone marrow manufacture red blood cells, platelets and various leukocytes. Platelets have hemostatic function, white blood cells can kill and suppress a variety of pathogens, including bacteria, viruses, etc.; some of the lymphocytes produce antibodies. Therefore, the bone marrow is not only a blood-forming organ, but also an important immune organ.

Spleen index:
Spleen is the body's largest lymphoid organ, located in the left upper abdomen. The main function of the spleen is filtering and storage of blood. Spleen is a crisp texture and a rich blood supply of organs; it is easy to break in the event of a strong external force. When the spleen ruptures it can cause serious bleeding. Spontaneous splenic rupture (SSR) is a rare but potentially life-threatening entity. It can be due to neoplastic, infectious, haematological, inflammatory and metabolic causes.

Thymus index:
Thymus (thymus) is an important lymphoid organ in the body. It's a ductless glandular organ at the base of the neck that produces lymphocytes and aids in producing immunity; it at-rophies with age which is closely associated with immune function. It is located in the chest before the mediastinum. During the late embryonic stage and birth, the human thymus weighs about 10 to 15 grams. With age, the thymus continues to develop and at adolescence it's about 30 ~ 40 grams. After puberty, the thymus shrinks to about 15 grams as we age.

Immunoglobulin index:
Immune globulin is a protein which has antibody function in humans. It's mainly made from human blood plasma. It's also found in other body fluids and tissue. Most of the immuno-globulin human plasma is present in the gamma globulin. Immunoglobulin can be divided into five types Immunoglobuli A, Immunoglobulin D, Immunoglobuli E, Immunoglobuli G, and Immunoglobuli G.

Respiratory immune Index:
The human respiratory system is the main gateway connected with the outside world. Pathogenic microorganisms and harmful substances can often lead to inflammatory diseases which enter into the respiratory tract in the air. There is lymphoid tissue located in the entire respiratory tract from the nasopharynx to the respiratory bronchioles and alveoli. Typical the lymph nodes are in the surrounding of the trachea and bronchi.

Gastrointestinal immune Index:

In recent years, with the development of immunology, people pay more attention to the relationship between the immune system and the digestive tract diseases. The digestive tract of a non-specific immunity include: full digestive tract from mouth to rectum mucosal barrier. This is where all decomposition of enzymes, bile, liver barrier, gas-trointestinal peristalsis and natural flora occur.

Mucosal immune Index:

The body defense mechanism has evolved to protect animals from invading pathogenic microorganisms and cancer. It is able to generate a diverse variety of cells and molecules capable of specifically recognizing and eliminating a limitless variety of foreign invaders. These cells and molecules act together in a dynamic network and are known as the immune system. Innate mucosal immunity consists of various recognition receptor molecules, including toll-like receptors, NOD-like receptors, and RIG-I-like receptors. These recognition receptor molecules recognize various invading pathogens effectively, and generate an immune response to stop their entry and neutralize their adverse consequences, such as tissue damage. Furthermore, they regulate the adaptive response in cases of severe infection and also help generate a memory response. Most infections occur through the mucosa. It is important to understand the initial host de-fense response or innate immunity at the mucosal surface to control these infections and protect the system. The aim of this review is to discuss the effects and functions of various innate mucosal agents and their importance in understanding the physiologi- cal immune response, as well as their roles in developing new interventions. Mucosal immune system is relatively independent of the systemic immune system. It is also inextricably linked with the systemic immune system. Mucosal immunity constitutes of two major functional areas: the immune induction site and parts of immune responses. Lymphocytes are part of the body's immune system. Mucosal immune system move continuously between the two major functional areas, accompanied by cell differentiation and maturation of their own.

It may be good to check this section if your client has a lot of health issues and ailments. If they have had surgeries and are on medications for various ailments, their immune system will be affected. This may give you an idea which immune system is affected. Please refer to the definition section of the book to get more detail.

HUMAN TOXIN ANALYSIS

Stimulating Beverage:

Stimulating beverages like pop have no or little electrolytes in them. If the person drinks these beverages after exercise, it is conducive to the body to add moisture after exercise and possibly results in the reduction of extracellular fluid osmotic pressure in the body. Due to the intake of a lot of fluid, to accelerate the further loss of intracellular electrolytes some people like drinking ice water after exercise. Although people feel cool after drinking ice water, the immediate drinking after exercise will stimulate gastrointestinal smooth muscle to cause gastrointestinal cramps and abdominal pain. Water temperature should be between 15 to 40 degree celsius, so the recovery process can be faster. The main ingredients of these stimulating beverages are sugar (or saccharin), pigment, carbohydrated water and carbohydrate dioxide. These stimulating beverages have little nutrition and high amount of calories. If the human body takes in excessive synthetic flavors and pigment, it is harmful. So we should drink less of these kinds of drinks. Juices is made from a variety of fruits, contain a variety of vitamins and sugars. Drinking fruit juice can supplement vitamins and inorganic salts in the body. The organic acids can regulate the acid-base balance of body fluid, stimulate the secretion of digestive juice, promote appetite and invigorate the spleen.

Electromagnetic Radiation:

I. What is electromagnetic radiation?: It is the interactive change of electric and magnetic fields generating electromagnetic waves; and the phenomenon of the air-launch or exposure of electromagnetic waves is called electromagnetic radiation. The electromagnetic radiation exceeding the safety limits causes electromagnetic pollution. At present, the electromagnetic pollution has become the first major pollution, being ranked before the sewage, waste gas and noise.

II. Electromagnetic radiation and physical health: studies have been done to see whether the electromagnetic field (50-60HZ) of industrial frequency impacts the physical health. Some countries have made a large number of surveys and statistical analysis and have obtained a surprising result: the probability of occurrence of human tumors is closely related to the low-frequency electromagnetic radiation.

III. Mechanism of electromagnetic radiation on the human body: The human body, being a conductor, can absorb electromagnetic energy. Under the action of electromagnetic field, the human body will cause thermal effects. The greater the strength of electromagnetic field, the more obvious the thermal effects are. In addition, it will interfere with the transmission of bio-electrical information of the human body.

IV. Harmful effects of electromagnetic radiation on the human body : electromagnetic radiation can widely impact the human health, and can change neurological, reproductive, cardiovascular and immune functions, eye vision, etc. The main symptoms include headache, dizziness, memory loss, inability of concentration, depression, irritability, women's menstrual disorders, breast cancer, skin aging, breathing difficulties, back pain and so on. The rate of the occurrence of leukemia in people exposed to electromagnetic radiation is 2.93 times higher than that of the healthy people, and the rate of occurrence of brain tumors is 3.26 times higher than that of the healthy people.

Tobacco / Nicotine:

When the content of nicotine reaches 1.2-1.8 milligrams, the mouse can be poisoned. The main harmful component of cigarette is tar, and nicotinamide is one of component in the tar. The nicotinamide is usually referred to nicotine, and the harm of nicotine is well known. In other words, whether cigarettes or their substitutes in which have nicotine have harm to the human body. As long as the nicotine is inhaled into the mouth, it will definitely harm the human body.

The Hazards of Smoking

I. Carcinogenesis

II. The effects on cardiac and cerebral blood vessels: Many studies suggest that smoking is the major risk factor of a number of cardiovascular and cerebrovascular diseases; all the incidental rates of coronary heart disease, hypertension, cerebrovascular disease and peripheral vascular disease of smokers are increased significantly. Statistics show that 75% of patients of coronary heart disease and hypertension have history of smoking. The incidence rate of coronary heart disease of smokers is 3.5 times higher than that of non-smokers, the mortality of coronary heart disease of smokers is 6 times higher than that of non-smokers, and the incidence rate of myocardial infarction is 2-6 times higher than that of non-smokers. By autopsy, we also find that the incidence rate of coronary arterioschlerosis of smokers is wider than that of non-smokers.

III. The effects on the respiratory tract: smoking is one of the main factors of chronic bronchitis, emphysema and chronic airway obstruction. Experimental studies have shown that long-term smoking can damage and shorten bronchial mucosal cilia and affect the clearance of cilia.

IV. The effects on the alimentary tract: smoking can generally cause gastric acid secretion to increase 91.5% than that of non-smokers, can inhibit the pancreas secreting sodium bicarbohydrate which results in the increase of duodenal acid load, thereby inducing ulcer. Nicotine in tobacco can reduce the tension of pyloric sphincter to make bile which leads to acid reflux, thereby weakening defensive factors of stomach and duodenum mucosa, prompting chronic inflammation and ulcers to occur, and delaying the healing of the original ulcers. In addition, smoking can reduce the tension of esophageal sphincter, easily leading to reflux esophagitis.

Pesticide Residue:

The original body of pesticides, toxic metabolites, degradation products and impurities left on the organisms, subsidiary agricultural products and environment, after use of pesticides are called as pesticide residues. People often only consider the residues of the original body of pesticides as pesticide residues and neglect toxic metabolite and the degradation products thereof. In fact, not only the original body is toxic, but also the chronic toxicity of its metabolites or impurities is equal to or more serious than the original. Pesticides can alter hormones to result in women's secretion disorders, male oligozoospermia and low sperm survival rate; after the pesticides enter the body, one part is converted by kidneys and livers or expelled to increase the workload of the body which causes diseases. Another part is combined with hemoglobin of blood to reduce its capacity for oxygen supply; and one part of fat soluble pesticides is deposited in the bodyfat.

Here, look at all of the various readings. If heavy metals are high, you may want to rec-ommend a heavy metal cleanse or a complete 5 phase cleanse like the one introduced by the Vital Heath Nutrition book.

Many clients may show a high reading in the stimulating beverage section as many people drink sodas, coffee, tea, gatorade, etc. This is an opportunity to introduce clients to more healthy natural beverages, such as herbal teas, organic juices, etc..

Many of us will have high readings for the electromagnetic radiation since we all use mobile phones, watch TV, use computers, etc. There are devices to protect you from electro-magnetic frequencies (EMF). These can be found online through various companies and sources. I acquired a stick-on blocker on my mobile phone to defrag the EMF coming from my phone into my body. If you are interested, contact me through my website and I can direct you to the supplier's contact information.

If your client smokes, or smoked in the past, they may have a higher than normal reading under the tobacco/nicotine section. Again, a cleanse program would benefit this client. Organs and tissues will still have a stored residue of nicotine and a proper cleanse may clean the tissues at a deeper level.

Many people will have higher than normal readings for Pesticide residue since most of us have consumed vegetables and fruits that were not organically grown. Much of vegetable and fruit produce are highly sprayed and these chemicals end up in our bodies. High levels can eventually have negative effects on our health. This is why cleansing once a year and also taking cleansing herbal supplements can help reduce residue buildup. Eating organic fruits

Helping people rebuild from the inside out.

and vegetables when you can obtain them also makes a difference in decreasing the amount of pesticides you ingest.

HEAVY METALS

Lead:

Blood lead levels is generally believed to be safe when it is in the range of 10 micrograms to 14 micrograms/liter; long term inhalation exposure to metallic lead or lead compounds in dust, can cause varying degrees of [lead poisoning] disease where the serum concentration is greater than 40 micrograms of lead/l. If it is inhaled too much it will harm the human

nervous system, heart and respiratory system, causing varying degrees of lead poisoning. Too much of it in the human body, can lead to interference with a variety of enzymes with a wide range of physiological effects on organisms and the organs of the body. The chances of lead poisoning in children are far higher than in adults.

Mercury:

Mercury ingested directly can absorb into the liver, brain, and the eye. It can also cause nerve damage mainly involving the central nervous system, the digestive system and the kidneys. In addition it will have a certain impact on the respiratory system, skin, blood and eyes. High levels of methylmercury in the bloodstream of unborn babies and young children can lead to causing the child less able to think and learn.

Cadmium:

Cadmium can cause irritation in the respiratory system. Long-term exposure can cause loss of the sense of smell and yellowing of the teeth. Cadmium compounds cannot easily be absorbed in the intestine, but can be absorbed into the body through breathing. Its accumulation in the liver or kidney can cause damage to the kidneys. Especially with the bone metabolic disruptions occur, resulting in osteoporosis, atrophy, deformation and a series of symptoms.

Chromium:

Chromium in nature mainly appears in the trivalent form of chromium and hexavalent chromium. Hexavalent chromium can harm people with slow chronic poisoning, which can be absorbed through the digestive tract, respiratory tract, skin and mucous membrane. It accumulates mainly in the liver, kidney and endocrine glands. It can also get into the respiratory tract which makes it easy to accumulate in the lungs. Hexavalent chromium can invade the body through the respiratory tract, then starts in the upper respiratory tract, causing rhinitis, pharyngitis, laryngitis and bronchitis.

Arsenic:

Arsenic invades the human body; it's discharged by the urine, digestive tract, saliva and breast. Its accumulation can contribute towards osteoporosis and has negative effects on liver, kidney, spleen, muscle, hair, nails and other parts. Arsenic in the nervous system stimulates the blood-forming organs. A small amount in the human body for a long time, has a stimulating effect on erythropoiesis. Long-term exposure to arsenic poisoning can cause cell and capillary poisoning, may also induce cancer.

Antimony:

Antimony is a silvery white metal, which can irritate the eyes, nose, throat and skin. Continuous exposure may damage the heart and liver function. Inhalation of high levels of antimony can cause symptoms including vomiting, headaches, breathing difficulties, and severe poisoning which can lead to death.

Thallium:

Thallium as a strong nerve poison. It can have damaging effects to the liver and kidney. Inhalation or oral consumption can cause acute poisoning. It also can be absorbed through the skin.

Many people will have a high reading in one or more of the Heavy Metal section. We are exposed to water that is fed through lead pipes, well water that may not always be totally pure because of pollutants seeping in through the ground, and chemicals in the air from all the emissions. We also have small amounts of arsenic, a trace element in plants, water and air. Some of the heavy metals come from plastics, paints, inks, and dyes used in many industries. In the environment we live in every day, as we drive our cars and inhale the smog, pollution, carbohydrate monoxide in the air, etc., we absorb some of these heavy metals. Again, a deep heavy metal cleanse would be advisable for clients with high readings.

BASIC PHYSICAL QUALITY ANALYSIS

Response Ability:

In the range of 59.786-65.424, it shows the adrenal function, compressive capacity and will-power are normal. The abnormality is when it shows the adrenal gland secretion is too low and the sentiment seems depressed and the response is slow. The number reading will be below 59.7.

Helping people rebuild from the inside out.

Mental Power:
In the range of 58.715-63.213, it shows the brain function and the vitality are normal. When the reading is below 58.7 it is in the abnormality range and it shows a weaker brain function, depression, insomnia, thinking and memory deterioration.

Water Shortage:
In the range of 33.967-37.642, moisture in the body is normal. When the reading is lower this is in the abnormality range which shows moisture in the body is too low, meaning the body is dehydrated and the person has a sense of thirst and fatigue. So it would be ap-propriate to supplement water. The long-term water shortage usually makes the skin dry and the person to age faster.

Hypoxia:
In the range of 133.642-141.476, it shows the oxygen content of the body's cells is normal. When the reading is lower it's in the abnormality range which means the oxygen content of the cells is low. Therefore the respiratory system is possibly abnormal, and there is an anemia trend. This could be due to lack of exercise. Also this can result in cell degeneration, memory loss and indigestion.

PH:
In the range of 7.350 - 7.450, it shows blood pH is normal. If pH is higher than 7.450, the body's blood is too alkaline. This is called alkalosis. Respiratory acidosis and alkalosis are due to a problem with the lungs. Metabolic acidosis and alkalosis are due to a problem with the kidneys.
Symptoms of alkalosis can include any of the following:
- Confusion (can progress to stupor or coma)
- Hand tremor.
- Lightheadedness.
- Muscle twitching.
- Nausea, vomiting.
- Numbness or tingling in the face, hands, or feet.
- Prolonged muscle spasms (tetany)

If the pH is lower than 7.350, the blood is acidic, and the body will start developing chronic diseases and generate the following symptoms:
1. fatigue, asthma and sleepyhead.
2. cold or diabetes, hypertension and gout.
3. obesity.

4. skin has more wrinkles and lacks of luster.

In the body, there are three kinds of mechanisms to regulate the PH value:

1. Blood protein.

2. Lungs expel carbohydrate dioxide to prevent the accumulation of carbohydrate.

3. Kidneys excrete acid-base and produce HCO- neutralization H + ion to regulate the PH value.

There are two main reasons that cause an acidic body:

1. High emotional stress.

2. Excessive intake of acidic foods.

The alkaline diet promotes the false idea that it is possible to change blood ph with diet. This is untrue, and major changes in blood ph could even be life-threatening. It is possible to change the ph of urine and saliva with diet. However, when the ph of these fluids changes, the ph of blood remains the same. Alkalinity means that something has a ph higher than 7. The human body is naturally slightly alkaline; with a blood ph of around 7.4. The stomach is acidic, which allows it to digest food. The ph of saliva and urine changes depending on diet, metabolism, and other factors.

Healthy physique is slightly alkaline, and people do not easily get sick. However, some research suggests that an alkaline diet may improve health, though not in the way that its supporters claim. Alkaline diets reduce a person's consumption of fatty and processed meats, and they encourage people to eat more fruits and vegetables. This offers several health benefits. In this section, it is advisable that you look at the Hydration levels and not focus on the other readings too much. The PH will only vary in small amounts from person to person.

ALLERGY ANALYSIS

Drug allergy index:

Drug allergy is due to drug-induced allergic reactions. Allergic reactions are a class of abnormal immune responses. Abnormal immune response, either too strong or too weak, the body is negative, it will cause a series of lesions; caused by the drugs effect is drug allergy. Usually the symptoms of the allergy are skin flushing, itching, heart palpitations, skin rashes, breathing difficulties and severe shock or death.

Alcohol allergy index:

Alcohol allergy is caused by the lack of the enzyme acetaldehyde of the body, and an external symptom of skin allergy reaction. The two necessary conditions to allergic reactions to alcohol are allergy and alcohol. Allergies are mostly because of the lack of acetaldehyde-converting enzyme which converts into acetic acid which metabolizes the alcohol. Hence this results in alcohol poisoning. These people will show a variety of allergy symptoms such as facial flushing, headaches, nausea, vomiting, and rapid heart rate. People who can drink large amounts of alcohol have enough of this enzyme in their body to metabolize the alcohol therefore no symptoms of poisoning occur.

Pollen allergy index:

The diameter of a pollen is generally about 30 to 50 microns. As they drift in the air they can easily be sucked into the respiratory tract. People who have pollen allergies have an allergic reaction after inhaling the pollen. The main symptoms of pollen allergy is sneezing, runny nose, watery eyes, nose, itching eyes and external auditory canal, also induced severe bronchitis, bronchial asthma, pulmonary heart disease (multiple in summer and autumn). The reason why the human body can cause pollen allergy is because the pollen is rich in protein. Some people are allergic to the protein component of the pollen.

Injection allergy

Certain percentage of people are allergic to injections including: penicillin, streptomycin, and other heterogeneous serum. 5% of the population to 6% of have injection allergies, and at any age, any dosage form, dose and with any route of administration. Therefore, the use of allergy testing should be done first and test results show negative before treatment.

Chemical products allergy index:

The raw materials of chemical fibered cloth are from coal, oil, gas and other high-molecular compounds or nitrogen compounds extracted. Some of these are likely to become allergic to the person when entering the body. It can easily lead to allergic dermatitis, causing itching, pain, swelling or blisters.

Paint allergy index:

Paint and other chemical products easily cause allergic reactions. However, the emergence of such symptoms is not necessarily due to substandard quality of paint, but by the decision of each person's body. Mainly two kinds of paint allergy symptoms exist.
1, the paint can cause allergic rhinitis: frequent hand-rubbing the nose, frequent sneezing, runny nose and smelling the paint fumes causing nausea and vomiting.
2, paint allergy can cause allergic dermatitis: the body, hands, etc., group of red points on the skin occur, become inflamed, and itchy.

Dust allergy index:

Inhalation of dust cause allergic reactions. When the dust is inhaled, allergy symptoms occur such as itchy nose, itchy skin, itchy eyes, wheezing and coughing. If you have asthma symptoms, you should go to hospital for treatment.

Smoke allergy index:
Some people are allergic to smoke inhalation. When the smoke fumes are inhaled, it can cause sneezing, runny nose, and sometimes can cause allergic dermatitis, causing itching, pain, swelling, or blisters.

Hair dye allergy index:
Contact with hair dye on the skin can cause: dermatitis, light performance of the scalp swelling, itching, burning, severe scalp, neck and facial swelling, blisters, streams of yellow water, or even purulent infection. Hair dye composition is called 'p-phenylenediamine' chemicals, The more frequent there is contact with hair dye, the more closely the chemicals attach themselves to the hair and scalp, the greater the harm to the body. Therefore greater the occurrence of hair dye allergy happening.

Animal fur allergy index:
Animal fur allergy is allergic to animal's fur is when after touching the fur there is a reaction. The allergic symptoms can be itchy nose, itchy skin, itchy eyes, wheezing and coughing.

Metal jewelry allergy index:
Jewelry allergy is a common cause of contact allergic dermatitis. Most jewelry allergy is caused by the metal nickel (see nickel allergy) which is used in the manufacture of precious metal alloys. More severe metal hypersensitivity reactions usually occur from prolonged exposure to a metal allergen through implants or metal ions that are inhaled or eaten. These reactions often cause chronic joint or muscle pain, inflammation, and swelling, leading to generalized fatigue and lack of energy.

Seafood allergy index:
Seafood allergy is due to the large number of heterogeneous seafood rich in protein, these mutant proteins directly or indirectly activate immune cells, causing the release of chemical mediators, and then produce a series of complex biochemical reactions. The interaction of Antibody-antigen, the human body shows symptoms of allergy.

Milk allergy index:
Milk allergy is allergic reaction to milk protein, and the symptoms can manifest as skin eczema, vomiting, diarrhea or abdominal pain and other symptoms. Milk protein molecules of the opposite sex sometimes can trigger allergic symptoms.
Go to this section to see if any of the allergies your client lists can be confirmed in the readings. They may not always show up as the scan has about a 70 percent accuracy reading.

Vital Health

SKIN ANALYSIS

Skin Free Radical Index:

It is inner poison which causes the greatest harm to human body. The skin's free radical is a product of the human body oxidation reaction. It is constantly generated and plays an important role in human aging process, pharmacological and toxicological effects. It also will damage the body's proteins, DNA, etc., and cause cell death or cancer. Skin will be loose, wrinkles form, and will it be dry.

Skin Collagen Index:

Collagen is a protein that serves as one of the main building blocks for your bones, skin, hair, muscles, tendons, and ligaments. "Collagen is what keeps our skin from sagging, giving us that plump, youthful look. It is a protein naturally produced in the body. It is the major insoluble fibrous protein in the extracellular matrix.

Your body naturally makes collagen, but this production decreases with age. "Starting in our mid-20s, we slowly begin to lose collagen," Dr. Aivaz says. "For women, we can lose up to 30% of our collagen production in the first 5 years of menopause." Because we lose collagen as we age, many are using collagen supplements as part of an anti-aging beauty regimen.

Dr. Aivaz says topical treatments like retinol and tretinoin are scientifically proven to promote collagen formation. Additionally, antioxidants such as vitamin C can reverse the inflammation that causes damage to the collagen in your skin.

"From what we know now, people are likely to get more benefit from retinol or vitamin C skin care products than from a collagen-containing cream," Dr. Aivaz says.

It is one of the most crucial raw materials in the biotechnology industry, and is the best biomedical material with huge demand. Its application includes biomedical materials, cosmetics, food industry, research purposes and the like. Collagen is slowly entering the field of cosmetic skin care now. Collagen is one of the major components of the human body's organizational structure. It is the most abundant protein, and accounts for about 25-33% of total body protein equivalent to 6% of body weight. It spreads to various tissues and organs throughout the body, such as: skin, bone, cartilage, ligaments, cornea, of the intima (inner layer of an artery or vein) , fascia, etc.. It is the main component that maintain morphology and structure of the skin and tissue organs. It is an important raw material for repairing injured tissues.

If collagen in the cortex is oxidized and fractured, its supporting role to skin is gone, thereby resulting in collapse of the heterogeneity and generating wrinkles.

Skin Grease Index:

Oily skin occurs because the sebaceous glands excrete its oil, and the skin presents a shiny look for long time. The skin is thick with large pores, and may generate acne and pimple easily. It is not easy to produce wrinkles. Facial make-up rarely lasts. Routine care should control skin oil secretion and maintain skin cleanliness regularly, thereby reducing blackheads, acne and pimple from occurring. Fresh and converged products should be selected for skin care, and exfoliation and deep cleansing should be intensified for weekly care. Moisturizing sunscreen should be used when exposed to the sun light to avoid skin aging. Products with thin texture and oil control efficacy should be selected for make-up.

Skin Immunity Index:

The immunity of the whole body should be first improved in order to improve skin immunity and prevent invasion of microorganisms such as viruses, bacteria, fungi and the like and skin allergic problems.

Specifically:

1. People should pay attention to eating more fungus (mushroom, cap fungus, black fungus, white fungus, golden mushroom, Agrocybe, and other common edible fungi), dark-colored vegetables and fruits (purplish cabbage, purple eggplant, purple grapes, sweet potato, etc.), food containing more zinc (livers of animals, seafood, apples, etc., zinc can enhance immunity, is beneficial for skin at the same time, and can reduce the sensitivity of the skin) in the aspect of eating.

2. People should do moderate exercise and have reasonable work and rest, and particularly should not stay up late, and should go to bed earlier.

3. People should maintain a healthy heart.

Skin Moisture Index:

Dry skin may be the biggest complaints of women. A recent survey shows that 60% of women are most concerned with dry skin problems, even more than the wrinkles. 70% of them claim that body skin is very dry in winter, and 40% of them have dry skin. (In summer, rates are respectively 34% and 15%).

Reasons for causing dry skin comprise:
1.   Aging
The skin's ability of retaining moisture declines, and sebum secretion will reduce with the increase of age.
2.   Insufficient sebum secretion
The surface of the skin is formed by sebum membrane, and can help skin maintain proper

moisture. Once the sebum secretion reduces, the secretion cannot meet the needs of manufacturing sebum membrane, and the skin becomes dry.

3.   Temperature lowering

The secretion of sebum and sweat will reduce rapidly in cold winter, but since the air is too dry, the skin moisture is gradually evaporated, the skin's surface becomes rougher, and the resistance will be weakened.

4.   Lack of sleep

Lack of sleep coupled with fatigue damage the body to a considerable extent, and the blood circulation will deteriorate. When the health is out of balance, the skin will have no energy and is prone to generate the dry and rough phenomenon.

5.   Weight loss

Extreme weight loss and partial eclipse also enable skin to become dry. When the skin cannot obtain sufficient nutrients, the skin cannot be fully flexible and will lose moisture, and thereby skin becomes dry and fragile. Dry skin disorder is also known as dry skin disease.

6.   Other reasons

When the indoor heating temperature is too high, bathing in water that's too hot, using harsh soap or detergent and endocrine changes. Also when women's estrogen levels decrease in the postmenopausal period.

Skin Moisture Loss:

Normal skin corneum only needs 10% -30% of moisture to maintain the skin's elasticity and softness. When the winter season comes, the air becomes cold and dry suddenly, temperature difference between day and night is great, the secretion of sebaceous glands and sweat glands reduces, and the water content of skin cells also declines sharply.

Skin Red Blood Trace Index:

Red blood trace is caused by telangiectasia (spider veins) in people's body, is often manifested in people's face, abdomen and buttocks as macular or linear red stripes, and is a common skin disease, and some people will experience a burning or an irritation feeling to different degrees.

Skin Elasticity Index:

Strong ultraviolet radiation easily causes skin keratosis and enables skin to lose elasticity, thereby causing premature aging. Skin elasticity can be improved through a healthier diet. Thereby making up for the skin damage caused by ultraviolet radiation. People should drink suitable amount of water. It is well known that the water content of human body tissue fluid achieves 72%, and the water content in bodies of adults is about 58% to 67%. Water in human body will be reduced continuously especially in summer under higher temperatures, thereby causing dry skin, reducing sebaceous gland secretion, and enabling skin to lose its elasticity. So it is important to drink sufficient amount of water every day. People should drink about an ounce of water per pound of their body weight everyday.

Skin Melanin Index:

Melanin can be widely found in human skin, mucous membranes, retina, pia mater encephali (delicate, vasculated fibrous membrane firmly adherent to the glial capsule of the brain and spinal cord), gall bladder and ovary. Melanin is composed of melanocytes. Skin melanocytes are mainly distributed in the basal layer of epidermis, and also can be found in our hair roots and outer hair sheath. Human epidermis may have about 2 billion melanocytes with the weight of about 1 g and are symmetrically distributed around the body with average 1560 per square millimeter. Melanocytes can synthesize and secrete melanin, therefore they are gland cells. However, the biosynthesis of melanin is very complex and is formed by tyrosinety-rosinase reaction in body colour (immature melanin). Disorder in any link of vitiligo melanin formation, transfer and degradation process can affect the metabolism, thereby resulting in changes in skin color.

Skin Horniness Index:

Skin is divided into epidermis, dermis and subcutaneous tissue. The skin epidermis is further divided into five levels of basal layer, spinous cell layer, granular layer, trans-parent layer and corneum from bottom to top in turn. Skin cells begin to grow from the basal layer and pass through the process of aging and death with the outward passage. Corneum is the final product of continuous regeneration of skin cells. When the skin surface corneum is thick, the skin will lose its luster, become gray, peel, wrinkle, and generate acne, etc.. The skin corneum formation cycle is about a month, so beauty experts pay attention to removing dead skin cells every 28 days.

For clients with skin problems, these readings may confirm some of their concerns. If their skin is too dry or aging too fast, then you may want to recommend some natural skin moisturizers found in the health food stores. I use a very good skin moisturizer called Pure Gar- dens. You can check it out at vitalcleanse.puretrim.com. It is a natural cream I personally use for dry patches on my skin during winter and also is a great antiseptic for cuts which heal twice as fast.

If a client has a severe skin condition, refer them to a doctor or a naturopathic doctor who specializes in skin remedies.

EYE ANALYSIS

Bags under the eyes:
Bags under the eyes are when the lower eyelid skin, subcutaneous tissue, muscle and the orbital septum relaxes. Also orbital fat hypertrophy occurs and the formation of the eye pocket protrudes.

Collagen eye wrinkle:
The main chemical component of the collagen fibers is collagen, a connective tissue fiber. This is loose connective tissue arranged in bundles with the fiber bundles branching out. Collagen and elastic fibers are woven together to form both toughness and elasticity. Both the organs and tissues withstand external traction, while maintaining a relatively fixed shape and location of loose connective tissue.

Dark circles:
Because of too many late nights, emotional instability, eye fatigue and aging, venous blood flow velocity is too slow. Also the dark circles are caused by lack of oxygen in red blood cells of eye skin. Furthermore, excessive venous carbohydrate dioxide and metabolic wastes accumulates. Chronic hypoxia creates the dark circles, and the formation of stagnant blood causes the eye pigmentation colour change.

Lymphatic obstruction:
Lymphatic obstruction for many reasons, can be divided into primary (causes unknown) and secondary. Secondary, includes inflammation, cancer, injury and from radiation therapy.

Sagging:
Because the fibers between the cells degraded over time, skin loses its elasticity; loss of subcutaneous fat, sagging skin and loss of support occurs. Skin and muscle relaxation also will make the skin loose.

Edema:
This is due to the effect of the variation of blood circulation. It becomes too late for the excess water to go out of the body through the excess waste water discharge system. Therefore, water retention in the capillaries, or the infiltration into the skin, produces the swelling edema.

Eye cell activity:
Cell activity is the cell's physiological state and function, reduce the temperature will slow

down the metabolism of cells, low temperature for a long time cause cell death, but the low temperature to a certain extent, also caused the cells in the suspension of respiration, but caused the cells to restore normal temperature, high temperature will lead to cell death.

Visual fatigue:

Visual fatigue occurs when we are engaged in work or study where we are reading books and computer screens up close a lot. Our eye experiences fatigue due to excessive use of our vision. Therefore, eye disease occurs from in close-in precision work, computer work or insufficient lighting. Many people suffer from myopia, hyperopia and other refractive errors. Patients with the usual symptoms are: blurred vision, some cannot write or read, dry eyes, dizziness, pain, and even severe nausea and vomiting.

If your client has a particular concern in regards to vision or eye disease or an eye ailment, some of the readings here may confirm the condition. Refer to the definition section for more detail.

COLLAGEN ANALYSIS

Eye:

When there is a lack of collagen in the eyes the following things happen, you experience dry eyes, fatigue, spontaneous tears, poor corneal transparency and lens opacity; eventually it can lead to cataracts and other eye diseases.

Tooth:

When the body lacks calcium, it pulls it from sources such as the teeth. This can lead to dental problems, including weak roots, irritated gums, brittle teeth, and tooth decay. Also, calcium deficiency in infants can delay tooth formation.

Hair and skin:

When collagen is low in the body the following things happen: dryness of hair, hair breaking off, hair loss, balding, bifurcation, increased dandruff; loose skin, cheeks, chin, eyes drooping. Also rupture of collagen fibers, increase in wrinkles; jaw ear contour is not clear, the formation of the accumulation of fat creating a double chin and ear; dry skin, sensitive skin, decreased flexibility, large pores and oily skin.

Endocrine system:

When Collagen is low in the body physical characteristics become obvious, amenorrhea (absence of menstruation in women), menstrual disorders, early entry into menopause;

dysplasia, breast sagging, breast hyperplasia, easy to cause breast cancer, could easily cause the masculine signs; male impotence, premature ejaculation, the male characteristics are not obvious.

Circulatory system:

When collagen is low in the body, vascular wall elasticity changes, the stability of blood pressure is affected: blood viscosity occurs, fatty liver, high blood cholesterol; slow blood circulation, the body absorbs poorly, weak metabolism, susceptibility to cardiovascular and Cerebrovascular diseases; memory loss, dizziness, forgetfulness and insomnia.

Digestive system:

Low Collagen causes decreased abdominal pressure causing organ posies, cardiac pumping, increased waist and abdomen size, flatulence; liver abnormalities, gallstones, mouth pain; poor secretion, diabetes, hematopoietic function weak, unbalanced, pernicious anemia and physical decline.

Immune system:

Low collagen causes slow lymphatic circulation leading to decreased immunity, easy infection of epidemic diseases, muscle pain, physical weakness and immune function is affected.

Motion systems:

Collagen levels in the body affect joint pain, decreased susceptibility to rheumatism, bone and joint flexibility; joint stiffness, bone hyperplasia; back meridian blockage, poor metabolism, back fat accumulation; easy to cause rheumatism, generalized muscle atrophy, bone deformation; cold hands and feet, numbness of the limbs, slow bone healing, loss of calcium; loss of collagen ligament strain, damage to joints and skeletal sites; fibrous tissue collapses, making the hips loose span sagging, deformation and fat increase followed by thickening.

Muscle Tissue:

Low collagen levels causes increase in fat mass, indurations (hardening of the soft tissue) of the cervical muscles, cervical spondylosis; back pain, shoulder tingling: connective tissue block, lactic acid accumulation in the nerve system, Yin hindering the reflex areas; poor muscle contractions, loss of energy, weak muscle pulling force and decreased muscle tone.

Fat Metabolism:

When the collagen is low metabolism decreases, fat accumulation occurs, more acidic; easily fatigued, prone to diabetes, high blood pressure resulting in liver and kidney failure.

Detoxification and metabolism:

When collagen is low susceptibility to accumulation of toxins in the body occurs, rough skin, constipation, physical obesity, acidic; a variety of visceral recession, kidney and spleen metabolic disorders, prone to nephritis, can lead to kidney failure; skin redness, itching skin, pain; body acne, various skin diseases, visceral dysfunction, mental decline and skin cancer.

Reproductive system:

When collagen is low it can lead to the shedding of the uterus, urinary incontinence, ovarian atrophy, low immunity, reproductive system; vaginal relaxation fold increase, dryness, women infertility, menstrual disorders and habitual abortion; male impotence, sexless; the phenomenon of stretch marks, loose anal muscle contractility, defecation pain, hemorrhoids, and pelvic pain.

Nervous system:

Collagen contains a large number of amino acids that are not only involved in the synthesis of new collagen, but also has affect on the central nervous inhibitory mechanism in the brain cells. The loss of collagen can cause memory loss, inability to concentrate, insomnia, anxiety, depression, irritability, anxiety, menopausal syndrome, poor response, nerve pain and so on.

Skeleton:

80% of the organic bone is collagen. Collagen loss will lead to decreased bone density and the formation of very fragile bones; will cause huge loss of calcium. Also will cause bone and joint pain, bone spurs, muscle atrophy, bones thickening, easy to cause bone cancer and leg paralysis, legs and feet are not flexible, osteoporosis, low glucosamine levels which support bones, easy to fracture, bone healing is slower, bone toughness declines and bones become brittle.

This section is worth looking at since collagen is one of the main substances in many parts of the body. Some of the conditions of your client may be due to the low collagen levels in that area of the body. There are actual natural collagen supplements available to recommend. One such supplement that helps restores collagen levels in the body is a product called Calorad, a liquid collagen which is consumed.

LARGE INTESTINE FUNCTION

Large intestine peristalsis function coefficient:
Large intestine has similar segmental motion and peristalsis with the small intestine, but its frequency is slower, this adapts the large intestine so one of its main function is absorbing

Tested Health Results Explained

CARDIOVASCULAR SYSTEM

BLOOD VISCOSITY

Definition: Blood viscosity is a measurement of the thickness and stickiness of an individual's blood.

Blood viscosity is an important blood property, and plays a key role in maintaining vascular homeostasis. Viscosity of the blood is affected by excess cholesterol and saturated fat, basically not the right diet, which causes them to circulate in the bloodstream like sludge and gradually deposit in the artery walls. Avoiding these unhealthy foods will help the blood to be clear in several days, but because most people consume these foods constantly, their blood is always polluted and viscous. The viscosity of the blood is also increased by stress since stressing causes the blood flow to increase and keep it in a fast flow for a longer period of time.

Levels:

High: Patients with high viscosity are prone to have Cerebrovascular accidents, such as stroke and other phenomena; coronary heart disease patients with high viscosity are prone to have myocardial infarction and so on.

If you want to prevent it, your doctor may recommend a heart-healthy diet or tell you about therapeutic procedures for decreasing blood viscosity: direct and indirect. Plasma exchange, phlebotomy, and rheopheresis are applied directly, whereas in indirect method, they regulate erythrocytes, platelets, and endothelial cells etc., which may have an effect on blood viscosity.

Low: If the blood viscosity readings are low, or too thin it can indicate anemia; also it can result in excessive bruising and bleeding.

Solution: Therefore, a heart-healthy diet includes fresh fruits and vegetables, 100 percent whole grains, healthy oils, low- or no-fat milk products, and healthy proteins. A heart healthy diet limits high-fat, high-cholesterol, and high-sugar foods.

Helping people rebuild from the inside out.   Vital Health

CHOLESTEROL CRYSTAL

Definition: A cholesterol crystal is a solid, crystalline form of cholesterol found in gallstones and arterioschlerosis.

A biochemical imbalance of lipids and bile salts in the bile can mediate precipitation of cholesterol leading to gallstones and gallbladder inflammation. Indeed, cholesterol monohydrate crystals form in supersaturated bile and they are regarded as a prerequisite for the development of cholesterol gallstones. Gallstones occurring in industrialized societies typically contain more than 70-90% cholesterol by weight, much of which is crystalline (A gallstone is a stone formed within the gallbladder out of bile components).

On the other hand, cholesterol crystals are a hallmark of arterioschlerosis, which is believed to be an early cause of atherosclerotic inflammation. Arterioschlerosis is a progressive disease starting with the accumulation of lipids, lipoproteins and immune cells in the arterial wall. Disease progression results in the narrowing of the arterial lumen due to continuous plaque growth. Therefore, cholesterol crystals are believed to induce inflammation.

Levels:
High: Increase is seen in primary high cholesterol blood, the aura of mild arterioschlerosis, blood stagnation type chest pain, phlegm congestion type, major cardio events and chest pain, etc.

Low: Reduction is seen in decreased immunity, malnutrition, cardiac insufficiency, Qi and Yin deficiency type chest pain, Yang Qi deficiency type chest pain, etc. Low levels of LDL cholesterol is rare but if it occurs there is an increased risk of cancer or hemorrhagic stroke. Symptoms of low cholesterol are hopelessness, nervousness, confusion, agitation, difficulty making a decision and changes in your mood, sleep, or eating patterns.

Prevention of cholesterol crystal formation might be achieved by lowering the plaque cholesterol load and enhancing the retrograde cholesterol transport, for instance by raising plasma levels of HDL ("good" cholesterol) or by increasing the expression of ABC transporters to promote HDL function. As low concentrations of HDL in the blood are among the most prominent risk factors for cardiovascular disease. HDL friendly food are, for example, olive oil, whole grains, fatty fish, avocados, etc.

Solution: You can reduce Cholesterol quickly by eating mainly fruits, vegetables, whole grains and beans. Keep your fat intake small, eat more plant sources of protein and stay away from refined flour foods. Even though the amount of exercise has been a matter of debate, most health organizations recommend a minimum of 30 minutes per day of moderate to vigorous exercise, such as walking, jogging, biking, few laps at the pool, some weight-lifting and some yoga five times a week. Also some vigorous aerobic activity for at least 20 minutes three times a week. This can raise your high density lipoprotein (HDL) which is the good cholesterol. It takes about It takes about three to six months to see lower LDL numbers through diet and exercise. Usually it takes longer to see the changes in women verses men.

BLOOD FAT

Definition: Blood lipids (or blood fats) are lipids in the blood, either free or bound to other molecules. They are mostly transported in a protein capsule, and the density of the lipids and type of protein determines the fate of the particle and its influence on metabolism.
The concentration of blood lipids depends on intake and excretion from the intestine, and uptake and secretion from cells.

Hyperlipidemia is abnormally elevated levels of any or all lipids or lipoproteins in the blood. Hyperlipidemias are divided into primary and secondary subtypes. Take note of two types of negative blood fat states in your clients. Primary hyperlipidemia is usually due to genetic causes (such as a mutation in a receptor protein), while secondary hyperlipidemia arises due
to other underlying causes such as diabetes. Lipid and lipoprotein abnormalities are common in the general population and are regarded as modifiable risk factors for cardiovascular disease due to their influence on arterioschlerosis.

Levels:
High: Increase in blood fat is seen in arterioschlerosis, idiopathic hyperlipidemia,
Other symptoms of high blood fat in the form of high levels of LDL and triglycerides can appear as chest pain (angina) or nausea and fatigue. Although you need triglycerides to supply your body with energy, having too much in your blood can Increase the risk of heart disease. About 25% of adults in the US have elevated blood triglyceride levels over 200 mg/dl. Some of the main causes of the high blood fat are obesity, uncontrolled diabetes, regular alcohol use and high-calorie diet.

Low: Decrease in blood fat is seen in low artery oxygen levels in the brain and dis-eases of the blood vessels in the brain. Also seen in decreased immunity.

Solution: The ways to reduce your lipid levels are (1) eat less fat, (2) exercise regularly and (3) lose weight if you weigh too much. If you smoke, stop smoking. If these steps do not lower your LDL level enough, your doctor may have you take medicine to take the fat out of your blood.

VASCULAR RESISTANCE

Definition: Vascular Resistance is the resistance that must be overcome to push blood through the circulatory system.

Levels:
High: If the resistance levels are higher than normal then it can be an indicator of cholesterol plaque build-up along the walls of blood vessels, which may also increase the blood pressure. Increase is in direct proportion to the length of blood vessels, and is in inverse proportion to the caliber of blood vessels. The increase of vascular resistance is seen in mildly elevated systolic and diastolic blood pressure, mild hyper-tension, insomnia with deficiency of heart and spleen, phlegm-heat internal confusion type insomnia, etc.

Low: Decline is seen in mildly declined systolic and diastolic blood pressure, mild hypotension, Yin deficiency and Huo exuberance type insomnia, etc.

VASCULAR ELASTICITY

Definition: The strength of artery expansion during ejection of blood from the heart. This occurs in the arterial system where the protein elastin forms an elastic mortar between the arrays of cells that line the arteries. There, the protein provides the stability that allows the vessels to expand and contract continuously as blood pulses along.

Healthy blood vessels are elastic, and elasticity helps to moderate blood pressure. Arterial stiffness increases with age and is a risk factor for cardiovascular disease and death. Studies have established that physical fitness can delay age-related arterial stiffness, although ex-actly how that happens is not understood. It is noted that people who keep themselves in shape often have a more flexible body, and they hypothesized that a flexible body could be a quick way to determine arterial flexibility.

Why would the flexibility of the body be a good indicator of arterial stiffness? In a study, researchers speculated on why this would be. One possibility is that there is a cause and effect: the stretching exercises that provide flexibility to the body may also slow the age-related stiffening of the arteries. The study found that arterial stiffness among middle age and older people was associated with trunk flexibility but was independent of muscle strength and cardiorespiratory fitness (as measured by performance on an exercise bike). In addition, they cited another recent study that found that middle age and older adults who began a regular stretch exercise program significantly improved the flexibility of their carotids, a major artery found in the neck.

Levels:
High: Increase is seen in mildly elevated systolic pressure (pressure when heart contracts and pumps blood out of body, mildly reduced diastolic pressure (pressure when heart relaxes and fills with blood), slightly high blood pressure, and a mildly increased pulse rate.

Low: A decrease in elasticity can indicate the arteries becoming clogged with fatty deposits (plaque), causing them to lose their elasticity and becoming narrower, therefore making the walls of the arteries thick and hard. This leads to mild arthro-sclerosis, coronary heart diseases, and chest pains due to lack of normal blood flow.

MYOCARDIAL BLOOD DEMAND

Definition: Myocardial oxygen demand is the amount of oxygen that the heart requires to maintain optimal function, and myocardial oxygen supply is the amount of oxygen provided to the heart by the blood which is controlled by the coronary arteries.

Since the heart operates solely under aerobic metabolism, myocardial mitochondria must maintain an abundance of oxygen to continue oxidative phosphorylation. Heart rate, contractility, and ventricular-wall tension are the three factors that determine myocardial oxygen demand. An increase in any of these variables requires the body to adapt to sustain adequate oxygen supply to the heart.

Heart rate is thought to be the most important factor affecting myocardial oxygen demand. With an increased heart rate, the myocardium must work harder to complete the cardiac cycle more efficiently. With a shortened cardiac cycle, the time spent in diastole decreases. Because diastole ends prematurely, the amount of blood that normally fills the ventricles decreases and oxygen-saturated hemoglobin is not allowed to reach the sub endocardium. Under optimal conditions, myocardial oxygen demand will equal myocardial oxygen supply; however, when there is structural damage from a plaque that impedes flow, there can be a mismatch between supply and demand that results in ischemia (Ischemia or ischaemia is a restriction in blood supply to tissues, causing a shortage of oxygen that is needed for cellular metabolism, to keep tissue alive.).

Levels:
High: When the myocardial blood demand is high, it could mean the heart rate is high as well which causes the myocardium to work harder to complete the cardiac cycle more efficiently.

Low: Low demand is seen in cardiac arrest where there is ineffective contraction of heart muscles. If its level is low, it can be from cardiac arrest where there is ineffective contraction of heart muscles.
Solution: This may correct itself once the client starts to exercise, lose excess fat and change their eating habits to more high anti-oxidant raw foods like fruits and vegetables.

MYOCARDIAL BLOOD PERFUSION VOLUME

Definition: The actual volume of blood per minute to the heart muscles.

Levels:
High: If the Myocardial Blood Perfusion readings are high, the damage to the heart is excessive. Coronary artery disease (CAD) has profound effects on the myocardial microcirculation If blood supply (blood flow) cannot meet the oxygen demand of the myocytes, myocardial ischemia ensues, and if uncorrected, infarction will occur.
        Low: If the Myocardial Blood Perfusion readings are low, indicates that there is low to no damage in the heart, but that the heart may be at risk of damage.

If the client has heart complications then please do not give any recommendations, unless you are a doctor. Refer them their doctor.

MYOCARDIAL OXYGEN CONSUMPTION (MOC)

Definition: Myocardial oxygen demand is the amount of oxygen that the heart requires to maintain optimal function, and myocardial oxygen supply is the amount of oxygen provided to the heart by the blood which is controlled by the coronary arteries.

High: When MOC is high, this means that there is higher heart rate, ventricular after load and preload (increased ventricular wall tension)

Low: The MOC readings will be low for clients who have some sort of coronary heart disease. Client with coronary artery disease will have decreased blood and oxygen supply to the myocardium. In this case, contractility will be diminished. Because the ventricle can no longer achieve adequate contraction, end systolic volume will increase.

Solution: This is where once you help a client to start to exercise and improve their diet the readings may increase over time. However, a healthy client who exercises and does a lot of cardio training will probably have close to normal readings, unless there is a structural problem with valves which some people are born with.

STROKE VOLUME (SV)

Definition: The blood volume output by the heart per beat.

5 Influence Factors:
(1) The effective circulating blood volume (BV): when the blood volume is insufficient, the returned blood volume is little, and the SV is reduced.
(2) The weakening of myocardial contractility: the contractility is low, and the pressure is low, so the ejected blood volume is less.
(3) The extent of ventricular filling: In range of myocardial elasticity, the greater the degree of filling is, the stronger the retraction is, and the SV is increased.
(4) The size of peripheral vascular resistance (PR). The PR is large, and then the SV is reduced; the PR is small, and then the SV is increased.
(5) Ventricle wall movement.
When the ventricle is contracted, the cardiac muscle is in coordinated movement. If the myocardial contraction is not coordinated, the SV is reduced. For instance, some patients with myocardial infarction have part of infarction, so the myocardial contractility is inconsistent and the SV is reduced. However, under normal circumstances, the ventricle wall movement cannot be abnormal.

Levels:
High: If the Cardiac Stroke Volume readings are high, then the heart is working too hard and can lead to heart damage and possibly stroke.
Low: If the Cardiac Stroke Volume readings are low, there is poor blood supply going

to the heart, which can lead to further complications if left unchecked.

LEFT VENTRICULAR EJECTION IMPEDANCE (VER)

Definition: Resistance of the left ventricle outflow channel

Influence Factors:

(1) The fact whether the outflow channel has lesion. Aortic stenosis and other conditions can make VER increase.

(2) The outflow channel has no lesion, while the emptying rate of aortic blood is slow, so VER is increased.

(3) The entire vascular resistance is large.

Levels:

High: The resistance of the left ventricle which pumps blood to the tissues cannot be too high. If it is too high, it can damage the heart and a stroke can occur.

Low: If it is too low, then not enough blood is going to the heart which can also create complications. Refer the client to their doctor if they have this kind of reading.

LEFT VENTRICULAR EFFECTIVE PUMP POWER

Definition: The contraction strength of an effective stroke of blood to the left ventricle.

This is the contraction strength of an effective stroke of blood to the left ventricle. If the readings for this are too high it can damage the heart and a stroke can occur. If it is too low, then not enough blood is going to the heart which can also create complications. Refer the client to their doctor if they have this kind of reading.

Levels:

High: If the Ventricular Effective Pump Power readings are high, it can lead to damage of the heart and possibly stroke.

Low: If the Ventricular Effective Pump Power readings are low, there is poor blood supply going to the heart, which can lead to further complications if left unchecked.

CORONARY ARTERY ELASTICITY

Definition: The degree of contraction of the artery that supplies blood to the heart.

Arterial elasticity has been previously linked to atherosclerotic vascular disease states. Serum uric acid level has been recently associated with increased arterial stiffness.

Levels:

High: This is the degree of contraction of the artery that supplies blood to the heart. If the reading is high, this means the vessels have weakened elasticity which can lead to heart failure and stroke

Low: If the Coronary Artery Elasticity readings are low, the vessels have become weak and can cause light headedness, dizziness, weakness, fainting and in the extreme cases, shock.

Solution: Again, if the readings of your client are very high or very low, refer them to their doctor. However, helping them with an improved diet of good fats, such as salmon, avocado and nuts, and cutting down on saturated fat foods, more plant based foods and sources of protein and having them start a mild exercise program, could make a positive difference in their heart issue.

CORONARY PERFUSION PRESSURE

Definition: Coronary perfusion pressure, also known as simply perfusion pressure, refers to the pressure gradient that drives coronary blood pressure, meaning the difference be-tween the diastolic aortic pressure and the left ventricular end diastolic pressure. It is a term used mainly in research concerning cardiac arrest.
Coronary flow is normally auto regulated so that within wide limits of changes in perfusion pressure (which is approximate to diastolic BP) blood flow to the heart remains constant. Thus, as perfusion pressure falls, the coronary arterioles dilate to maintain flow; under basal conditions a five-fold increase in coronary flow can occur, i.e. a flow reserve of five.

Levels:

High: If the Coronary Perfusion Pressure readings are high, it indicates that the vessels have become less elastic which can lead to a risk of strokes, heart attacks, heart failure and renal failure.

Low: If the Coronary Perfusion Pressure readings are low, it indicates that the vessels have become weak and can cause light headedness, dizziness, weakness, fainting and in extreme cases shock.
Solution: Again, this is probably due to high plaque buildup in the arteries and a change in nutrition and a proper exercise program could make a huge difference.

Gastrointestinal Function

PEPSIN SECRETION COEFFICIENT

Definition: Pepsin is secreted as pepsinogen and released into the stomach. It is a digestive enzyme that partially breaks down proteins found in protein sources such as eggs and meats. The remaining digestion of the protein occurs in the small intestines. Pepsinogen is converted to pepsin by hydrochloric acid in the stomach.

Levels:
    High: If the pepsin secretion coefficient levels are high, then it indicates an excess of pepsin, and an excess of pepsin in the stomach can cause irritation of the mucosa.
    Low: If the pepsin secretion coefficient levels are low, then it indicates a state of hypochlorhydria (Note. stomach unable to produce hydrochloric acid).

Solution: If a client has a low pepsin reading and you know by their food score results and health conditions that they suffer from weak digestive issues, a good recommendation is to have them eat more raw vegetables to help them digest protein better in the stomach. The extra enzymes of the raw vegetables and fruit juices can make a difference in these cases. Also, taking high quality extra probiotic and enzyme supplements can totally make a difference.

GASTRIC PERISTALSIS FUNCTION COEFFICIENT

The muscles in your digestive system move food forward in a wavelength motion called "peristalsis". Gastric peristalsis grinds the food for further processing as well as the role of gastric juice to make food into a gruel kind of chime, and then the chime is ejected into the small intestines in batches through the pylorus. The time of processing food in the stomach is different. The processing time of carbohydrate foods is shorter than that of protein foods, and the processing time of fat and oily foods are the longest, so we can have less of an appetite after eating fatty foods.

Peristalsis can be blocked, slower than it should be, or not a strong enough contraction to move food forward. Bowel-related reflexes can become weaker or less effective due to:

- reliance on laxatives
- restricted eating patterns
- eating disorders, such as anorexia or bulimia
- use of narcotics
- anesthesia
- irritable bowel syndrome

There may be other reasons for weaker muscles as well. Sometimes the cause is even as simple as not having enough fiber in your diet.

High: This is when the person's peristalsis moves too much, too fast and this is known as rapid gastric emptying. The most common cause of rapid gastric emptying and dumping syndrome is surgery of the stomach or esophagus. Types of surgery that may lead to dumping syndrome include

- Bariatric surgery, such as gastric bypass surgery and gastric sleeve surgery. These operations help people lose weight.
- Esophagectomy, which is surgery to remove part of the esophagus. Doctors use this surgery to treat problems of the esophagus, such as esophageal cancer NIH external link and Barrett's esophagus.
- Fundoplication, which is surgery to sew the top of the stomach around the esophagus. Doctors use this surgery to treat gastroesophageal reflux disease and hiatal hernia.
- Gastrectomy, which is surgery to remove all or part of the stomach. Doctors use this surgery to treat stomach cancer NIH external link and peptic ulcers.
- Vagotomy, which is surgery to cut the vagus nerve in the stomach so that the stomach makes less acid. Doctors use this surgery to treat peptic ulcers.

Rapid gastric emptying sometimes occurs in people who have not had stomach surgery. For example, rapid gastric emptying may occur in people who have

- Recently developed diabetes, especially type 2diabetes
- Pancreatic exocrine insufficiency, a condition in which the pancreas doesn't make enough of certain enzymes, causing problems with digestion
- Duodenal ulcers

Low: Low reading can indicate the client has poor nutrition, not enough fiber and not enough exercise. Therefore they have a slow, weak peristalsis action.

Solution: Eating more raw vegetables, fresh organic vegetable juice, whole grains, more fiber, consume extra probiotic with a very high count of bacteria and strong enzyme supplements can increase the peristalsis action in a person's digestion.

GASTRIC FUNCTION ABSORPTION COEFFICIENT

The gastric gland secretes a transparent acidic gastric juice, and the gastric gland of an adult can secrete 1.5-2.5 liters of gastric juice each day. Gastric acid, gastric juice, or stomach acid fluid comprising a mixture of substances, including pepsin and hydrochloric acid, secreted by glands of the stomach. Its principal function is to break down proteins into polypeptides during digestion. The acidic environment caused by the gastric acid can help the small intestines absorb iron and calcium.
Gastric acid is produced by cells in the lining of the stomach, which are coupled in feedback systems to increase acid production when needed.

The absorption in the human digestive system is mainly a function of the small intestine, some absorption of certain small molecules nevertheless does occur in the stomach through its lining. This includes:
• Water, if the body is dehydrated
• Medication, such as aspirin
• Amino acids
• 10–20% of ingested ethanol (e.g. from alcoholic beverages)
• Caffeine
• To a small extent water-soluble vitamins (most are absorbed in the small intestine)

The parietal cells of the human stomach are responsible for producing intrinsic factor, which is necessary for the absorption of vitamin B12.

High: High reading can indicate that the client may have acid indigestion, eats food too fast, not enough chewing. Also an impaired function of the vagus nerve or an overactive thyroid gland can also cause the gastric absorption function to be too fast. Another cause can be Celiac disease where the person cannot digest gluten which is a protein in wheat, barley, rye and other grains. Also people who have had surgery for abdominal ulcers, anti-reflux surgery or gastric bypass may have this condition.

Low: Low reading can mean low absorption of proteins from the foods being digested in the stomach. Also lack of fiber in the diet, certain medications such as opioid pain relievers, some antidepressants, and high blood pressure and allergy medications, can lead to slow gastric emptying and cause similar symptoms. For people who already have gastroparesis, these medications may make their condition worse.

Solutions: A solution for this is a diet that emphasizes natural, unprocessed fruit and vegetables which can kick-start digestion and help make you more regular unless you have IBS, gastroparesis or other chronic gastrointestinal condition.

The following things can improve absorption in the stomach:

Eat a variety of foods in one meal

Pair vitamin C-rich foods with Iron

Include healthy fats with each meal

Take lots of high quality strong probiotic and enzyme supplement

Avoid drinking tea, water or any liquids while eating; drink water or liquids at least one hour before or one hour after any meal or snack.

SMALL INTESTINE PERISTALSIS COEFFICIENT

Once processed and digested by the stomach, the milky chime is squeezed through the pyloric sphincter into the small intestine. Once past the stomach, a typical peristaltic wave only lasts for a few seconds, travelling at only a few centimeters per second. Its primary purpose is to mix the chime in the intestine rather than to move it forward in the intestine. Through this process of mixing and continued digestion and absorption of nutrients, the chime gradually works its way through the small intestine to the large intestine.

High: This is when the peristalsis is working too much, too fast which will cause diarrhea, loose watery stool and client will have a sense of urgency to eliminate.

Low: Low reading indicates that the small intestine could have abnormalities in the muscle and are usually associated with diseases such as scleroderma. These connective tissue disorders may cause the intestine to balloon out in places so that the contractions of the muscle are not able to move the contents downstream.

Also the following diseases cause intestinal dysmotility: systemic Lupus erythematosus, amyloidosis, neurofibromatosis, Parkinson's disease, diabetes, scleroderma, thyroid disorders, and muscular dystrophies. Certain medications can also cause intestinal dysmotility.

The symptoms will be slow digestion, bloating, hardened dry stool, painful, difficult elimination and constipation.

Solutions: Delayed or slower bowel movements can be caused by a lack of fiber in your diet. A diet that emphasizes natural, unprocessed fruit and vegetables should kick-start your digestion and make you more regular. Also not drinking enough good water that is pure and absorbs well affects bowel movement and transit time of your stool. Therefore dehydration is a huge reason for such problems as acidic issues in the bowels, constipation, gas, bloating, etc..

Examples of foods that supports your digestion include:

- almonds and almond milk
- prunes, figs, apples, and bananas
- cruciferous vegetables such as broccoli, cauliflower, Brussels sprouts, and bok choy
- flax seeds, sunflower seeds, and pumpkinseeds

Limiting dairy, which can be difficult to digest, and cutting out bleached, processed, and heavily preserved baked goods may also help. Ice cream, potato chips, and frozen meals have little to no fiber and should be avoided.

Cutting back on coffee, which dehydrates the digestive system, could also be a way to balance out your bowel movements. Also consider adding two to four extra glasses of water to your daily routine.

Taking probiotic supplements has been shown to improve the transit time and regularity of bowel movements.

Light exercise can direct your blood to circulate through your abdomen. For some people, this gets the system going. Consistent exercise may impact your lazy bowel symptoms by keeping your digestive system turned "on" and engaged. Some yoga poses may even help relieve constipation.

SMALL INTESTINE ABSORPTION FUNCTION COEFFICIENT

The small intestine is the part of the gastrointestinal tract between the stomach and the large intestine where much of the digestion of food takes place. The primary function of the small intestine is the absorption of nutrients and minerals found in food.

Low: Usually the readings in most people will be low in this section particularly in people who eat foods that are high density, low water content and low enzymes. These foods are common especially in a western culture. The absorption rate will be slow due to the quality of the foods being low. Therefore, if there is refined sugar and preservatives in the food there can also be inflammation as well occurring in the small intestine.

Also another factor that may cause malabsorption or weak absorption is: damage to the intestine from infection, inflammation, trauma, or surgery, prolonged use of antibiotics. other conditions such as celiac disease, crohn's disease, chronic pancreatitis, or cystic fibrosis.

Liver Function

PROTEIN METABOLISM

Definition: Protein metabolism denotes the various biochemical processes responsible for the synthesis of proteins and amino acids, and the breakdown of proteins by catabolism. The steps of protein synthesis include transcription, translation, and post translational modifications.

After digestion, proteins are absorbed by the small intestine and then sent to the liver for metabolism in order to manufacture a variety of proteins according to the body's needs.

In many cases, you will have low readings in this section, meaning that either the liver is not functioning well or the foods which are processed are too high in fat, causing higher toxicity in the liver which can contribute to the liver malfunctioning.

Levels:

If the protein metabolism level is high, it can indicate improper digestion of food in the stomach, which can cause stress on the liver. A high total protein level could indicate dehydration or a certain type of cancer, such as multiple myeloma, that causes protein to accumulate abnormally.

If the protein metabolism level is low, it indicates a malfunctioning liver or kidney. Also could mean protein is not being digested or absorbed properly.

ENERGY PRODUCTION FUNCTION

Definition: After carbohydrate digestion, the liver will carry the sugars to various parts of the body that are in need of it and convert the glucose into glycogen for storage. After fatty foods are digested, the liver will convert fat into energy.

The readings in this section may be low because the client has not consumed enough carbohydrates in their diet. The readings in the liver function will change over time as the person changes their eating habits or consumes more or less protein, fats and carbohydrates which will give different readings here. However, the low readings of this section can be used to make suggestions to your client for consuming proper amounts of healthy carbohydrates and protein. Following proper food combining principles will help them not to overwork the liver's function.

Levels:
If the energy production function level is high, it indicates an overconsumption of carbohydrates.
If the energy production function level is low, it indicates a carbohydrate-deficient diet.

DETOXIFCATION FUNCTION

Definition: During the metabolic and digestive process, food will produce some toxins. The liver and detoxifying enzymes will detoxify harmful substances (alcohol, ammonia) into harmless substances (e.g. water, urea and carbohydrate dioxide) to be excreted out of the body.
If this reading is high, you may want to recommend your client improve their diet, reducing alcohol consumption and processed foods, which both stress the liver's detoxification function. Eventually, the liver can breakdown from high amounts of alcohol consumption, which is what happens to alcoholics.
A low reading is not good either because it means the liver is not getting rid of the toxins fast enough; hence further health issues can occur.

Levels:
If the detoxification function level is high, it indicates the liver is working extra hard and cannot keep up with the demands of the body.
If the detoxification function level is low, it indicates the liver is not getting rid of the harmful substances properly, which can lead to a number of health issues.

BILE SECRETION FUNCTION
Definition: Bile is the final product of metabolism in the liver, which aids in the digestion of fat and aids the body to absorb fat-soluble vitamins A,D,E and K.
Levels:
If the bile secretion function level is high, it can result in the gallbladder temporarily shutting down, which can begin to form gallstones. Also this mean too much bile is being secreted which causes the gallbladder to stop functioning temporarily. This then leads to formation of gallstones. Therefore, if you have a client who already has passed gall stones and their diet is poor, you may want to suggest they follow a lower fat diet so their gallbladder does not shut down too much, creating more stones in their gallbladder.

If the bile secretion function level is low, it can result in the gallbladder not functioning properly, poor digestion which can lead to high cholesterol. Furthermore, a low reading means not enough bile is being secreted to look after digestion of fat which can lead to higher cholesterol. You may suggest, if you are looking at nutrition with a client, that they start consuming raw vegetable juice, with some black radish in the juice. The black radish stimulates the gall- bladder to produce more bile which can help in digesting fat in the diet, therefore de-creasing bad LDL cholesterol levels.

LIVER FAT CONTENT

Definition: If the liver fat content is more than 5% of wet weight, the liver can be classified as a fatty liver. Also, if 1/3 of liver cells per unit area on a liver biopsy have liquid droplets under a microscope, that can also be classified as a fatty liver.

Levels:
If the liver fat content is high, it can indicate the following: the person may not experience any symptoms. If it is moderately high, the person may experience symptoms such as loss of appetite, fatigue, nausea, vomiting, diarrhea, liver pain, left shoulder and back pain.

If the liver fat content is low, it can indicate malabsorption of nutrients because of not enough bile being secreted from the liver to breakdown the fats in the food consumed.

Solution: If the reading is high in the liver fat content, then a diet low in fat is necessary for the client. Also a weight loss program should be implemented if the client is heavy. A cleanse will also bring the fat down in the body and in the liver as well.

Helping people rebuild from the inside out.

Gallbladder Function

SERUM GLOBULIN

Definition: Globulins are proteins in the fluid part of the blood (serum). They are produced in the liver and others are made by the immune system. They contain most of the antibodies of the blood.

Levels:
If the serum globulin level is high, it can indicate immune hyperactivity of body, cirrhosis, hepatitis, liver Qi stagnation type hypochondriac pain, liver and gallbladder damp-heat type hypochondriac pain
If the serum globulin level is low, it can cause mild liver and gallbladder discomfort. It can also be a sign of liver or kidney disease.

TOTAL BILIRUBIN

Definition: Bilirubin is a yellow pigment that is in blood and stool. It is made in the body when red cells are broken down. The breakdown of old cells is a normal and healthy process. All the bilirubin in the blood is called total bilirubin.

Levels:
If the total bilirubin is high, it indicates hemolytic jaundice (yellowing of the skin or the whites of your eyes).
If the total bilirubin level is low, it can indicate low immunity and potential liver and gall bladder diseases.

ALKALINE PHOSPHATASE

Definition: Alkaline phosphatase is a protein found in all body tissues.
Levels:
If Alkaline Phosphatase levels are high, it can indicate intrahepatic and extrahepatic obstructive jaundice, mild or moderate hepatitis, liver and gallbladder damp-heat hypochondriac

pain.
If Alkaline Phosphatase levels are low, it can indicate mild hepatitis, sub-health status and low immunity.

SERUM TOTAL BILE ACID

Definition: Bile acids are contained in bile, which help digestion and absorption of fats and fat-soluble vitamins in the small intestine.

Levels:
If serum total bile acid levels are high, it can indicate the person can be developing obstructive jaundice or cholestalsis and, perhaps because of their inherent detergent activities, it can cause hepatocyte injury. Thus, increased bile acid levels in hepatocytes may account for some of the liver damage in cholestatic liver diseases.
If serum total bile acid levels are low, people may exhibit various signs or symptoms, including: Vitamin deficiencies, specifically of fat-soluble vitamins such as A, D, E, and K. Jaundice, the classic yellowing of the skin and whites of the eyes. Stunted or abnormal growth. Diarrhea.

BILIRUBIN (DIRECT)
Definition: Bilirubin attached to sugar is called direct bilirubin

Levels:
If bilirubin levels are high, it can indicate obstructive jaundice, liver cell jaundice
If bilirubin levels are low, it can indicate hemolytic jaundice.

Pancreatic Function

INSULIN

Definition: Insulin is a protein whose role is to reduce blood sugar. It promotes the liver, muscle and adipose tissue to take up glucose from the blood.

Levels:
If the insulin levels are high, it can indicate heart problems. High readings of insulin can signal heart problems. With proper nutritional changes, cleanses, weight-loss and exercise your client can greatly correct their heart problems in a lot of the cases. A Chinese assessment can be done where there are Chinese herbal formula supplements that help strengthen the heart.

If the insulin levels are low, Low readings usually indicate your client is possibly on their way to becoming a diabetic. Look at all the other assessment results, such as the food score and the hormone assessment sheet, to confirm your conclusion. If you see that the client eats a lot of sugar, refined high carbohydrate foods and they are overweight, then they may well be on their way to becoming a type 2diabetic.

PANCREATIC POLYPEPTIDE

Definition: Pancreatic Polypeptide (PP) is a protein secreted by the pancreas whose function is to self-regulate the secretion activities of the pancreas. It also has effects on gastrointestinal secretions and hepatic glycogen levels.

Levels:
If the PP levels are high, it can indicate diabetes, pancreatic tumor with secretory function; cirrhosis (liver disease), chronic kidney disease; such as the pancreatic polypeptide cell hyperplasia, myocardial infarction, severe heart failure, non-cardiogenic shock and duodenal ulcer.
If the PP levels are low, it can indicate obesity and chronic pancreatitis (inflammation of the pancreas).8

GLUCAGON

Definition: Glucagon is a hormone, which raises blood glucose levels. The pancreas releases glucagon when blood glucose levels are low. Once glucagon is released, it stimulates the liver to convert glycogen into glucose, which is then released into the blood. Glucagon also stimulates the release of insulin so glucose can be used by insulin-dependent tissues. Therefore, glucagon and insulin work as a feedback system to keep blood glucose levels optimal.

Levels:
If the glucagon levels are high, it can indicate insulin-insensitive diabetes and pancreatic glucagonoma.
If the glucagon levels are low, it can indicate congenital and cell deficiency.

Kidney Function

LYSOZYME ACTIVITY

Definition: Lysozyme in the urine and serum of kidneys is an antimicrobial enzyme, which aids in the killing of microorganisms such as bacterial species by breaking apart the cell structures of the bacteria.

Levels:
If the lysozyme activity is negative, it indicates normal activity.
If the lysozyme activity is positive, it can indicate damage of kidney tubules, nephropathy, renal injury, mild sclerosis of the renal arteries and decreased immunity.

URINE PROTEIN
Definition: The amount of protein present in urine, which is used to aid in the evaluation and monitoring of kidney function and to help diagnose early kidney damage and disease.

Levels:
If the urine protein levels are negative, it indicates normal activity.
If the urine protein readings are positive, it can indicate proteinuria (proteins present in urine)9 and edema.

UREA NITROGEN

Definition: The blood urea nitrogen is a measure of the amount of nitrogen in the blood in the form of urea, which is also an indication of kidney function. Urea is a substance secreted by the liver and removed from the blood by the kidneys.

Levels:
If urea nitrogen levels are negative, it indicates normal activity.
If the urea nitrogen levels are high its positive, it indicates a moderate to severe kidney failure. If the kidneys have trouble excreting urea, it can be due to conditions such as dehydration and shock or may be due to acute or chronic disease of the kidneys.

URIC ACID

Definition: Uric acid is a waste product in the blood due to breakdown of compounds called purines. Most uric acid dissolves in the blood passes through the kidneys and leaves the body in the urine that you pass. Excess uric acid can cause crystals to form in the joints and cause gout.

Levels:
If uric acid levels are Low it's a negative number, it indicates normal activity.
If the uric acid levels are High it's a positive number, it can indicate acute and chronic nephritis, edema and gout.

UROBILINOGEN

Definition: Urobilinogen is a colour-less product due to breakdown of bilirubin. Bacteria in intestines cause the breakdown. Some urobilinogen is reabsorbed and excreted by the kidney.10

Levels:
If urobilinogen levels are Low it is a negative number, it indicates normal activity
If urobilinogen levels are High it is a positive number, it indicates or leads to jaundice, edema, billiary tract infection, hemolytic jaundice and hepatocellular jaundice.

Lung Function

VITAL CAPACITY

Definition: The volume change of the lung between a full inhalation and maximal exha-la-tion.

Levels:
If the vital capacity is higher than 3529 the high end of normal range, it indicates that the vital capacity is increased, which is seen in mild upper respiratory tract infections, and mild chronic bronchitis, phlegm retention in the lung and coughing.
If the vital capacity is lower than 3348 the low end of normal range, it can indicate reduced lung capacity, which can result in mild chronic bronchitis, lung cough, and chronic obstructive pulmonary emphysema.

TOTAL LUNG CAPACITY
Definition: The volume of air contained in the lungs at the end of maximal exhalation.

Levels:
If total lung capacity is higher than 4782 high end of normal range, it can indicate mild emphysema and shortness of breath.
If the total lung capacity is lower than 4301 low end of normal range, it can indicate extensive lung tissue lesions, chronic bronchitis and upper respiratory tract infection.

AIRWAY RESISTANCE RAM

Definition: Airway resistance assessments evaluate airway responsiveness, evaluation of sites of airflow resistance or closures, characterization of the type of lung disease.

Levels:
If the airway resistance is higher than 1.709, it can indicate chronic obstructive pulmonary emphysema, chronic bronchitis, bronchial asthma, lung and kidney deficiency.
If the airway resistance is lower than 1.374, it can indicate upper respiratory tract infection,

mild bronchial pneumonia and retention of phlegm in the lung.

ARTERIAL OXYGEN CONTENT

Definition: Blood gas analysis is performed on blood from an artery. It measures the partial pressures of oxygen and carbohydrate dioxide in the blood, oxygen content, oxygen saturation, bicarbohydrate content and blood Ph.11

Levels:
If arterial oxygen content is higher than 20.012, it can indicate weak lungs.
If arterial oxygen content is lower than 17.903, it can indicate early symptoms of bronchial asthma and whopping cough.

Brain Nerve Function

STATUS OF BRAIN TISSUE BLOOD SUPPLY

Definition: Cerebral blood flow is the blood supply to the brain in a given time. In an adult, the CBF is 750 mm per minute.

Levels:
If the brain tissue blood supply levels are high, a condition known as hyperemia can raise intracranial pressure, which can damage delicate brain tissue
If the brain tissue blood supply levels are low, ischemia can occur or in severe cases, brain tissue death.

CEREBRAL ARTERIOSCHLEROSIS

Definition: A blockage of the brain's arteries that results from thickening and hardening of the artery walls. Strokes can result and aneurysms can be produced. A rupture of an aneurysm (localized enlargement of artery walls as a result of the weakening of an artery wall) can produce bleeding (hemorrhage).

Levels:

If the cerebral arterioschlerosis levels are high, it can indicate hardening or blockages are forming in the cranial arteries.

If the cerebral arterioschlerosis levels are low, there is generally nothing to be concerned about.

FUNCTIONAL STATUS OF CRANIAL NERVE

Definition: Cranial nerves are nerves that are located in the brain. In humans, there are 12 pairs of cranial nerves.

Levels:
If the cranial nerve levels are high, it indicates a poor diet and lots of stress.
If the cranial nerve levels are low, there is generally nothing to be concerned about.

CRANIAL NERVE SENTIMENT INDEX

Definition: Sentiment is one's attitude toward objective things and the reflection of when other people's needs are satisfied. Sentiment can be divided into two categories: positive and negative. Positive sentiment can bring an enhancement of immune function and general health which can improve one's quality of life. Negative sentiment (being upset, sadness, anxiety, resentment etc) is detrimental for mental and physical health.

Levels:
If Cranial Nerve Sentiment Index levels are high, it indicates stress, anxiety and poor mental health.
If Cranial Nerve Sentiment Index levels are low, it indicates sadness and apathy.

MEMORY INDEX
Definition: Memory index reflects the strength of a person's memory. There are two types of memory: auditory and visual.12

Levels:
If memory index levels are high, it often indicates impaired short term memories.
If memory index levels are low, it indicates impaired long term memory.

David S. Lee *Helping people rebuild from the inside out.* Vital Health

Bone disease

LUMBAR FIBER PROTRUDING DIMENSION

Definition: Lumbar Fiber Protruding Dimension shows the lumbar (lower part of back) fiber cycle and how it protrudes toward one side of the body or protrudes near the side.
If the Lumbar Fiber Protruding Dimension levels are indicating anything than No Di-rection, then it is not in normal healthy range.

SHOULDER MUSCLE ADHESION

Definition: Shoulder Muscle Adhesion shows the extent of shoulder inflammatory lesions in elderly people.

Levels:
If the Shoulder Muscle Adhesion levels are higher than <u0.2, it indicates that there is a shoulder scarring or muscle adhesion to a certain degree.
If the Shoulder Muscle Adhesion levels are lower than u0.2, it indicates that the illness is lighter in elderly individuals or there is an absence of body disease.

LIMBS CIRCULATION LIMIT

Definition: Limbs Circulation limit shows the limit of stiffness or activities in the micro-circulation of blood in the limbs as a result of external factors.

Levels:
If the Limbs Circulation Limit readings are greater than 1, it indicates that the microcircula-tion of blood in the limbs are impaired which makes the limbs more susceptible to disease.

AGE OF LIGAMENT

Definition: Age of ligament is an integrated parameter from the above three indicators, in which the results are between 10% and40%.

Levels:
If the age of ligament levels is high, it can indicate to some degree, degenerative diseases or aging.

If the age of ligament levels are low, it indicates that the physique and human immunity are compromised.

Bone Mineral
Density Analysis

OSTEOCLAST COEFFICIENT

Definition: Osteoclasts are a type of bone cell that removes bone tissue by the process of removing its mineralized matrix and degrading the organic bone (organic dry weight is 90% collagen). This process is known as bone reabsorption. The osteoclast coefficient is the imbalance between the bone and bone formation.

Levels:
If the osteoclast coefficient level is high, it indicates that healthy bone is being broken down faster than new bone being formed.
If the osteoclast coefficient level is low, it generally indicates no concern.

AMOUNT OF CALCIUM LOSS

Definition: The rate of the loss of calcium in the bones.

Levels:
If the calcium loss levels are high, it indicates that the body is losing calcium at a higher and faster rate than normal
If the calcium loss levels are low, it generally indicates no concern.

BONE HYPERPLASIA
Definition: Bone hyperplasia is the bone state. During the process of bone growth, development and function completion of bone, some parts lose the normal shape. Due to different structure and parts of bone across the body, bone hyperplasia is in various forms.

Levels:
If bone hyperplasia levels are high, it indicates a greater than normal deficiency in bone min-

eral.
If bone hyperplasia levels are low, it generally indicates no concern.

OSTEOPOROSIS

Definition: Osteoporosis is a disease where bones become weak and fragile. Without prevention and treatment, osteoporosis can progress without any pain or symptoms until a fracture occurs.

Levels:
If osteoporosis levels are high, it indicates osteoporosis.
If osteoporosis levels are low, it generally indicates no concern.

BONE MINERAL DENSITY

Definition: Bone mineral density reflects the strength of bone, and is a good diagnosis of osteoporosis, and can also predict the probability of fracture occurrence.

Levels:
If the Bone Mineral Density factor readings are high, it indicates that bone mineral density is deteriorating.
If the Bone Mineral Density factor readings are low, it generally indicates no concern.

Rheumatoid Bone Disease

DEGREE OF CERVICAL CALCIFICATION

Definition: Cervical calcification determines the rate of calcification of the cervix. No calcification means there is an absence of hyperplasia (increase in the amount of bone tissue as a result from cell proliferation). Basic calcification means the rate of hyperplasia is 30% and calcification means the rate of hyperplasia reaches over 70%.

Levels:
If the Degree of Cervical Calcification level is high, it indicates that cervical calcification is accelerating.
If the Degree of Cervical Calcification level is low, it generally indicates no concern.

DEGREE OF LUMBAR CALCIFICATION

Definition: Lumbar calcification determines the rate of calcification of the lumbar. No calcification means there is an absence of hyperplasia (increase in the amount of bone tissue as a result from cell proliferation). Basic calcification means the rate of hyperplasia is 30% and calcification means the rate of hyperplasia reaches over 70%.

Levels:
If the Degree of Cervical Calcification level is high, it indicates that lumbar calcification is accelerating.
If the Degree of Cervical Calcification level is low, it generally indicates no concern.

RHEUMATISM COEFFICIENT

Definition: Broad Rheumatism is a group of diseases that impact bone joints and their surrounding soft tissues, such as muscle tendon, fascia etc. Narrow rheumatism refers to a set of acute and chronic inflammatory diseases of connective tissue triggered by upper respiratory tract due to Group A bacterial Streptococcus.

Levels:
If the rheumatism coefficient level is high, it indicates that rheumatism is starting to become a serious concern.
If the rheumatism coefficient level is low, it generally indicates no concern.

Blood Sugar

COEFFICIENT OF INSULIN SECRETION

Definition: Insulin is a protein hormone which is secreted by specialized cells from the pancreas known as β-cells. Insulin primarily functions to lower levels of blood sugar. The coefficient of insulin secretion determines the balance of insulin and glucose.

Levels:

If the coefficient of insulin secretion levels is high, it indicates that calories are converting to fat which can lead to obesity.

If the coefficient of insulin secretion levels is low, it indicates metabolic disorders caused by poor insulin secretion, including sugar, protein, water, fat and electrolytes.

BLOOD SUGAR COEFFICIENT

Definition: The blood sugar coefficient is the relation of glucose absorption and blood sugar levels.

Levels:

If the blood sugar coefficient level is high, it can indicate hyperthyroidism, lack of insulin (seen in Type 1 and Type 2 diabetes), adrenal cortex hyperactivity, central disease, anterior pituitary and adrenal cortex hyperactivity, vomiting, diarrhea, and fever. It is normally seen in 1 to 2 hours after meals and after glucose injection during emotional stress.

If the blood sugar coefficient level is low, it can be due to hunger, excessive insulin secretion (insulin excess disorders and excess insulin injected or oral hyperglycemic drug), hypothyroidism, malnutrition, acute liver injury, genetic enzyme deficiency, excessive loss of blood sugar. After physiological activities such as sports, the blood sugar coefficient level can also drop.

URINE SUGAR COEFFICEINT

Definition: Urine sugar coefficient is the relation of glucose absorption and urine sugar levels.

Levels:

If the Urine Sugar coefficient level is high, it can indicate physiological glucosuria caused by consuming a large amount of a food consisting of high carbs at once. Late pregnancy of women who are lactating can have this condition. It can also indicate renal glucosuria, in which the kidneys are reabsorbing glucose at a much reduced rate. It can also indicate diabetes and hyperthyroidism.

If the urine sugar is low which is a normal state, the body can reabsorb the fluid of the body before it leaves the kidney to be excreted as urine.

Human Toxin

HEAVY METAL

Definition: Heavy metals include hexavalent chromium, Lead, Arsenic and Mercury.

Levels:
If the heavy metal factor readings are high, it indicates an elevation in one or more of the afore mentioned heavy metals. Hexavalent chromium can lead to bronchial asthma, skin erosion, ulcers and allergic dermatitis. Chronic exposure can lead to respiratory cancer. Lead compounds can mainly affect the nervous system, kidneys and blood system of the human body. It can also affect children's mental development and cause renal dysfunction. Chronic arsenic poisoning can cause fatigue, weakness, convulsions, skin damage, keratinisation, hair loss, cancer and pigment deposition. Mercury on the human body causes headaches, dizziness, numbness and pain.
If the heavy metal factor readings are low, it is not a concern.

STIMULATING BEVERAGE

Definition: Stimulating beverages include soda, pop and energy drinks which have few or no electrolytes.

Levels:
If the Stimulating Beverage readings are high, it indicates an excess of artificial stimulants inside the body.
If the Stimulating Beverage readings are low, it is generally not a concern.

ELECTROMAGNETIC RADIATION

Definition: The combination of electric and magnetic fields produce what is called electromagnetic radiation.

Levels:

If the Electromagnetic Radiation levels are high in the body, it indicates that electromagnetic radiation is present in the body. EMR can impact and change neurological, reproductive, cardiovascular and immune functions and eye vision. Symptoms include headache, memory loss, inability to concentrate, dizziness, depression, irritability, breast cancer, skin aging, breathing difficulties, back pain etc. The rates of leukemia and brain tumors are much higher in people who do not protect themselves from EMR.

If the Electromagnetic Radiation levels are low, it generally indicates no concern.

TOBACCO/NICOTINE

Definition: Tobacco is prepared from leaves of the tobacco plant by changing their colour and reducing their chlorophyll. Tobacco contains a stimulant called nicotine, which is a risk factor for a lot of diseases, especially the heart, liver, lungs and many cancers.

Levels:
If tobacco levels are high, in indicates an elevated level of nicotine in the body.
If tobacco levels are low, it generally is not of a concern.

PESTICIDE RESIDUE

Definition: Pesticide residue evaluates the toxic pesticide in the body. Pesticides can alter hormones and can have a affect on women's secretion disorders, oligozoospermia (low sperm concentration in males), and low fertility rate. Once the pesticides enter the body, one part of it is converted by the kidneys and liver or expelled to cause a work overload of other body organs which cause disease. Another part of pesticides is combined with hemoglobin of blood which reduces its oxygen carrying capacity. One part of fat-soluble pesticides is de-posited in the body fat.

Levels:
If the Pesticide Residue levels are high, it indicates an increased level of pesticide residue in the body.
If the Pesticide Residue levels are low, it generally indicates no concern.

Trace Elements

CALCIUM

Definition: Calcium is the most abundant mineral in the body which is found in certain foods, medications and included in many dietary supplements. Calcium is required for

muscle contraction, expansion and contraction of blood vessels, enzyme and hormone secretion, and transmitting impulses through the nervous system. 99% of calcium is stored in bones and teeth where it supports their structure.

Levels:
If calcium levels in the blood are high, irregular heartbeats and extremely low blood pressure can result. If one allows the condition to worsen, it can lead to loss of consciousness or a feeling of confusion. High calcium levels can also lead to depression, abdominal pain, kidney pain, and possibly kidney stones and kidney disease. Too much calcium can be as a result of consuming calcium forms that the body cannot assimilate.
If calcium levels in blood are low, calcium deficiency and osteoporosis – a weakening of the bones that puts people at high risks for fractures. Calcium deficient people can also suffer from dental problems and hypertension.

IRON

Definition: Iron is essential to human body function. Iron is a key part of many proteins and enzymes that maintain good health. Iron is essential component in the transport of oxygen around the body. It is also essential for cell growth regulation and differentiation. Two-thirds of iron in the body is found in hemoglobin, which is the protein in red cells that carry oxygen to tissues. Iron is also found in proteins that store iron for future use and that transport iron in blood.

Levels:
If iron levels are high, it can lead to toxicity and potential death.
If iron levels are low, it indicates iron deficiency which can ultimately result in anemia.
Symptoms of anemia include fatigue, decreased immunity and poor work performance.

Helping people rebuild from the inside out. Vital Health

ZINC

Definition: Zinc is an important mineral that participates in a wide range of metabolic activities. Zinc is required in healing injuries, necessary for growth and development, hair growth, insulin production, immunity, smell, taste and fertility. Zinc is also important during pregnancy to ensure the fetus undergoes proper growth and development.
Levels:
If Zinc levels are high, it can cause nausea, vomiting and diarrhea.
If Zinc levels are low, it can indicate zinc deficiency which can include some of the following symptoms: behavioral and sleep disturbances, dandruff, diarrhea, acne, skin lesions such as eczema, delay in wound healing, hair loss, long nails, growth retardation, hyperactivity, inflammation of nail cuticles, inflammatory bowel disease, loss of appetite, loss of sex drive, mild anemia, loss of the taste or smell sense, pre-menstrual syndrome, toxaemia in pregnancy and post-natal depression, reduced fertility, skin dryness and rashes, white spots on finger-nails, and poor nail growth.

SELENIUM

Definition: Selenium is a trace mineral that is essential to good health but only required in small amounts. Selenium is needed to make important antioxidant enzymes, which help prevent cell damage, which can further lead to heart diseases and cancer. Other uses of selenium are to help regulate thyroid function and play a role in immunity.

Levels:
If selenium levels are high, it can lead to nausea, vomiting and skin lesions.
If selenium levels are low, it can possibly lead to heart problems and deterioration of joint tissue.

Prostate

DEGREE OF PROSTATIC HYPERPLASIA

Definition: A non-malignant (non-cancerous) enlargement of the prostate gland, which is common in older men. Prostatic hyperplasia occurs in men in their 30s and commonly causes symptoms after 50.

Prostate gland grows in size in prostatic hyperplasia. It can possibly compress the urethra which can impede the flow of urine from the bladder through the urethra to the outside. Common symptoms include difficulty in letting the urine stream, a high urge to urinate and more severe problems such as urinary tract infections. Also complete blockage of the urethra which can lead to kidney injuries can occur.

Levels:
If the Degree of Prostatic Hyperplasia levels are high, then one of the more aforementioned conditions above is present which can cause an increased risk for cancer.

If the Degree of Prostatic Hyperplasia levels are low, it generally indicates no concern.

DEGREE OF PROSTATIC CALCIFICATION

Definition: A precursor of prostate stones is known as fibrosis, which is a scar left by prostate inflammation. The stones will give rise to bacteria, so fibrosis (prostate calcification) is also a reason for recurrent prostatitis and cannot be ignored. Prostate calcification is manifested as urinary obstruction or bowel obstruction and even inflammation of connective tissue. Some patients may have testitis and epididymitis.

Levels:
If the Degree of Prostatic Calcification levels are low, it generally indicates no concern.
If the Degree of Prostatic Calcification levels are high, then one of the more aforementioned conditions above is present which can cause an increased risk for cancer.

PROSTATITIS SYNDROME

Definition: Prostatitis syndrome is an inflammation of the prostate gland in men. Symptoms include urinary urgency, frequent urination, dysuria, urethral burning, rectal and perineal pain, fever and aversion to cold and discomfort to the lower abdomen. Prostatitis can be caused by bacteria, fungi, parasites and viruses.

Levels:
If the Prostatitis Syndrome levels are low, it generally indicates no concern.
If the Prostatitis Syndrome levels are high, then one of the more aforementioned conditions above is present which can cause an increased risk for cancer.

Male Sexual Function

TESTOSTERONE

Definition: Testosterone is a hormone primarily responsible for growth and male sex and reproductive organs, which includes the penis, testicles, scrotum, prostate and seminal vesicles. It helps in the development of secondary male characteristics such as musculature, bone mass, fat distribution, hair patterns, vocal cord thickening, and laryngeal development.

Levels:
If testosterone levels are high, people are more likely to engage in risky and irresponsible behaviour.
If testosterone levels are low, a decreased sex drive and sexual dysfunction occurs also with a decline in physical energy, strength and stamina, mental aggressiveness, more aches and pains in the bones and joints and less initiative.

GONADOTROPIN

Definition: Gonadotropin has a role to aid in the maturation of the reproductive organs, such as the testis and ovary. When puberty starts, the concentration is increased to promote the sexual maturation, thus, they have an important role in sexual development.

Levels:
If the Gonadotropin levels are high, mood swings and aggression can result.
If the Gonadotropin levels are low, it can lead to genital dysplasia and sexual growth retardation.

ERECTION TRANSMITTER

Definition: Erection transmitter (Erection conduction) depends on a complex interaction of neural, vascular, psychological and endocrine factors. Testosterone has an important role in this process. Neurotransmitters are also involved in starting and maintaining a better penis erection which includes dopamine and nitric oxide.

SKIN

SKIN FREE RADICAL INDEX

Definition: All cells in the body produce what's called free radicals. Free radicals are cells that are missing an electron in its outer shell. Therefore, those cells will attack other healthy cells to grab an electron to fill its outer shell. This is called oxidative damage, which causes aging of biological organisms. Collagen, the building block of our skin, is damaged as a result of those free radicals attacking other healthy cells. Free radicals have been associated with skin cancer, and premature skin aging.

Levels:
- If the skin free radical index levels are high, it indicates an increased production of
- collagen.
- If the skin free radical index levels are low, it indicates the collagen level is low or poor.

SKIN COLLAGEN INDEX

Definition: Collagen is a biological polymer which is one of the main components of the body's organizational structure, is the most abundant protein and accounts for 25-33% of total body protein which is equivalent to 6% body weight. Collagen is found in skin, bone, cartilage, ligaments and cornea. It is the main component of scaffolding cells, tissues and organs, including the skin, and an important raw material in repairing damaged tissues. With- out collagen, the body would fall apart literally.
Collagen generally diminishes as we age, and our body's ability to replace damaged collagen diminishes, which leads to wrinkles.
Levels:
- When collagen level is high: Collagen is a protein that makes up connective tissues, such as the skin. When you have too much collagen, your skin can stretch, thicken, and harden.
- Systemic scleroderma affects the skin, as well as blood vessels and internal organs.
- Scleroderma causes your body to produce too much collagen.
- When collagen level is low: three main things will lower your collagen levels: sun-light, smoking, and sugar. Too much exposure to ultraviolet light makes its fibers un-ravel. This can lead to sun damage, such as wrinkles. Many of the chemicals in cigarette smoke can damage it, which can make skin sag and wrinkle

Helping people rebuild from the inside out.   **Vital Health**

SKIN GREASE

Definition: Also known as oily skin: sebaceous glands (secrete an oily and waxy matter), excrete strongly, and the skin appears shiny. The skin is thick with large pores, which may generate acne and pimple easily. Care should be taken to control oil secretion to prevent these unpleasant protrusions.

Levels:

- When skin oil levels become high even after the oily skin is cleansed it feels greasy within hours. Breakouts are also more likely because the sebum mixes with dead skin cells and gets stuck in your pores. The causes of oily skin include genetic, environmental, and life-style factors.
- Also hormones and oily skin seem to go hand in hand. Androgens are the hormones mostly responsible for oil production, and sometimes they can fluctuate, stimulating an increase in sebum production. This often happens during puberty, just before
- menstruation, during pregnancy and during menopause.
- When skin oil levels become low the skin becomes dry. Dry skin isn't usually serious. In most cases it's caused by factors like hot or cold weather, low moisture in the air, and soaking in hot water. You can do a lot on your own to improve your skin, including using moisturizers and avoiding harsh, drying soaps.
- Occasionally, a dry skin problem can be a sign of an internal medical condition. For instance, aging may inherently make people more prone to dry skin. In addition, eczema, psoriasis, diabetes, hypothyroidism, and malnutrition are all associated with dry skin.

SKIN IMMUNITY INDEX

Definition: Prevent invasion from microorganisms such as viruses, bacteria, fungi etc. The skin is not only a physical barrier between external and internal environments actively protecting from stress caused by injury, microbial treat, UV irradiation, and environ-mental toxins. For a long time, skin was envisioned only as a static shield separating from external milieu. The concept of skin immunity and skin-associated lymphoid tissue was introduced by Streilein (1983) and this concept, although with caution, has been further extended to nominate skin as a peripheral lymphoid organ (Egawa and Kabashi-ma 2011; Ono and Kabashima 2015). Immune system within the skin is located in both major structural compartments: epidermis and dermis and consist of several important types of immunocompetent cells. Main skin-resident immune cells, Langerhans cells (lcs) together with melanocytes that produce melanin, occupy epidermis, whereas the other types of immune specialized cells such as various dendritic cell (dcs) subpopulations, macrophages, and several T cell types reside in deep- er layer—dermis. The effectiveness of the skin immune system strongly depends on the close interplay and communication between immune cells and the skin environment, e.g., neigh- boring keratinocytes and fibroblasts. Direct functional success of the skin immunity depends also on the flexibility of dermal vessels and the lymph nodes that drain the skin.

Levels:
- When skin immunity index is high it will protect against sunburn, infections, injury pro- vides surveillance for emerging cancers, removes damaged cells, and prevents undesirable autoimmune reactions against cell proteins.
- When skin immunity index is low the skin will manifest as mottled dyspigmentation, sagging of the skin, wrinkling, fragility, loss of elasticity, easy bruisability, accumulation of precancerous lesions, and epithelial and melanocyticneoplasms.

Solution: Maintain a healthy heart, Moderate exercise; have reasonable work and rest Eating more fungus (mushroom, white fungus, golden mushroom and other common edible fungi), dark coloured vegetables such as purplish cabbage, purple eggplant, purple grapes, sweet potato), food containing more zinc (livers of animals, seafood, apples etc)

SKIN MOISTURE INDEX

Levels:
- When skin moisture is low it's because of the following things:
- Aging
- Insufficient sebum secretion because sebum helps maintain skin moisture
- Low temperature cause sebum and sweat secretion to decrease in winter. Moisture will be evaporated due to the dry air, causing more rough skin
- Lack of sleep which results in lack of energy and is prone to generate dry skin
- Weight loss due to lack of nutrients causes dry skin
- Indoor temperature heating is too high, bathing in hot water
- When skin moisture is high it is because of Moisture in skin is retained by lipid, natural moisturizing factor (NMF) and ceramide. All these components are found in the
- peripheral of the stratum corneum (skin's outer layer).

Solution: A good goal is to drink about one ounce of pure ionized reduced alkaline water per one pound of your bodyweight every day. Add water-rich foods such as watermelon, straw- berries, and cucumber. These can help give your skin and body the hydration it needs to look and feel amazing!

SKIN MOISTURE LOSS

Definition: Abnormality is primarily in winter season where the air is dry and the temperature difference between the day and night is great, therefore, the secretion of sebaceous and sweat glands decreases.

SKIN RED BLOOD TRACE INDEX

Definition: Red blood traces on skin is caused by dilated blood vessels (telangiectasia), which can be seen on face, abdomen and buttocks, a common skin disease. Some people will show burning and irritation to varying degrees.

SKIN ELASTICITY INDEX

Definition: UV radiation causes skin to lose elasticity, which causes premature aging. Compensation can be achieved by drinking suitable amount of water. Water dehydration will also cause the skin to lose its elasticity.
Levels:
Skin elasticity is high when you can stretch it out and it comes back to original shape.
Skin elasticity is low mean there is loss of skin elasticity which is known as elastosis. Elastosis causes skin to look saggy, crinkled, or leathery.

Areas of the skin exposed to the sun can get solar elastosis. These parts of the body may look more weathered than those protected from sun exposure. Solar elastosis is also referred to as actinic elastosis.

SKIN MELANIN INDEX

Definition: Skin melanin index is widely found in human skin, mucous membranes, retina, gall bladder, ovary etc. Disorder in any link of melanin formation, transfer and degradation process can affect metabolism, thus, resulting in skin colour changes.

Levels:
- When the skin level of melanin is high your skin gets darker.
- When the skin level of melanin is low your skin gets lighter and it causes patches of light

skin.

SKIN HORNINESS INDEX

Definition: Skin Horniness Index is the ability for the outermost part of the skin (epidermis) to keep the body protected from the outside environment. The epidermis also has another duty: to keep the skin hydrated and prevent the body from losing water.
Levels:
When it is too high the skin is tough and calloused
When it is too low the skin will have luster, less wrinkles, smoother

Gynecology

Female Hormone:
Female Hormone is mainly produced by the follicule and corpora luteum. It stimulates the adolescent girl's genitalia, vagina, fallopian tubes and uterus to develop and grow, stimulate the emergence of female secondary sexual characteristic, affect the metabolism, and has a promotion role for adolescent development and growth.

Gonadotropin:
The role of gonadotropin is mainly to promote maturation of the reproductive organs, such as ovary. If the amount of gonadotropin secretion is insufficient, it may lead to genital dysplasia and sexual growth retardation. The gonadotropin is divided into luteinizing hormone and follicle stimulating hormone. Before the puberty, the concentration of the hormone is very low. When the puberty starts, the concentration is increased to promote the sexual maturation.
Thus, they have an important role in sexual development. The role of follicle stimulating hormone is mainly to promote the ovary to produce ovum, and the role of luteinizing hormone is to promote ovulation and produce estrogen and progesterone. Women's menstrual cycle
is regulated by them. Before the puberty, the amount of gonadotropin secretion is less and has no difference between day and night. After the puberty starts, the amount of secretion is significantly increased during sleep. During the mid-puberty, a lot of gonadotropin is secret-ed during sleep and waking. During the post puberty, the concentration of gonadotropin is increased greatly and is almost close to the adult level.

Levels:
* High: It is not known what the effects are of having too much gonadotrophin-releasing hormone. Extremely rarely, pituitary adenomas (tumours) can develop, which increase

production of gonadotrophin leading to overproduction of testosterone or estrogen.

- Low: In women the failure of adequate pulsatile gonadotropin secretion leads to failure of egg development or ovulation, initially at intermittent cycles; oligomenorrhea ensues before the onset of amenorrhea and estrogen deficiency. Symptoms of gonadotropin
- deficiency frequently bring to attention the possibility of evolving hypopituitarism if these individuals are not undergoing regular endocrine screening.

Prolactin:

The concentration of blood prolactin is also closely related to the sexual behavior. At present, it is known that the gonadotropin secreted by the female pituitary can adjust the level of ovarian secretion of estrogen and lutin and play a decisive role in sexual activity of female. Prolactin can act on the hypothalamus in feedback to reduce the estrogen secretion to cause vaginal dryness and difficult sexual intercourse and aggravate female sexual pain or discomfort, and thereby the female gradually generates fear for sexual life to lead to reduced sexual desire. For instance, before and after the menstrual period, women's sexual desire is relatively reduced due to the decline of sex hormone level. In another example of women who enter old age, due to the gradual shrinkage of ovarian, the sex hormone level is significantly decreased, so the apathy for sexual desire can be caused. After these older women supplements sex hormones, it can recover their sexual requirements. These can prove that sex hormones are closely related to the sexual desire. In clinic, some infertile women have the problems of inhibited sexual desire or apathy for sexual desire due to difficult sexual intercourse caused by vaginal dryness. The examination also finds that the concentration of prolactin in blood of these infertile women is elevated. Prolactin can act on the hypothalamus in feedback to reduce the estrogen secretion to cause vaginal dryness and difficult sexual intercourse and aggravate female sexual pain or discomfort, and thereby the female gradually generates fear for sexual life to lead to reduced sexual desire. Therefore, the concentration of blood prolactin is also closely related to the sexual behavior.

Levels:

- High: High prolactin levels interfere with the normal production of other hormones, such as estrogen and progesterone. This can change or stop ovulation (the release of an egg from the ovary). It can also lead to irregular or missed periods. Some women have high prolactin levels without any symptoms.
- Low: The condition of having too little prolactin circulating in the blood is called hypo-prolactinaemia. This condition is very rare and may occur in people with pituitary under activity. A decrease in the amount of prolactin secreted can lead to insufficient milk being produced after giving birth.

Progesterone:

Lutein is mainly produced by corpora luteum in the ovary, so it is also known as progesterone. The lutein is secreted by the placenta after pregnancy. Lutein usually exerts the role on the basis of the role of estrogen, and provides for the planting of the fertilized ovum in the womb and ensuring pregnancy. For instance, lutein makes the endometrium convert into a secretory phase from the growth phase to facilitate embryo implantation and cause the uterus not be easily excited, thereby ensuring that the embryo has a 'quieter' environment. On the basis of the role of estrogen, lutein promotes galactophore development and prepares the conditions for lactation after pregnancy. Lutein also has the heating function to raise the basal body temperature by 1 degree or so after ovulation. The body temperature is transitorily lowered before ovulation and rises after ovulation, so the change of the basal body temperature is used as one of the symbols determining the ovulation date in clinic; lutein can make the internal women 'suterus muscle relax and the activity reduce to be beneficial to the growth and development of fertilized ovum in the uterine cavity; lutein promotes endometrium of the proliferative phase to be converted to secrete its intima to prepare for the fertilized ovum nidation; lutein promotes the mammary acinar development and inhibits ovulation, so women during pregnancy do not ovulate and do not produce menstruation.

Levels:
- High: High levels of progesterone are associated with the condition congenital adrenal hyperplasia. However, the high progesterone levels are a consequence of and not a cause of this condition. Also, high levels of progesterone are associated with an increased risk for developing breast cancer.
- Low: Females who have low progesterone levels may have irregular periods and struggle to get pregnant. Without this hormone, the body cannot prepare the right environment for the egg and developing fetus. If a woman becomes pregnant but has low progesterone levels, there may be an increased risk of pregnancy loss.

Vaginitis coefficient:

Vaginitis is a kind of inflammation of the vagina mucosa and submucous connective tissue, is a common disease of gynecological outpatients. The vagina of normal healthy women has a natural defense function when pathogens intrude, as a result of the anatomical and biochemical characteristics of the vagina. When the natural defense function of the vagina breaks down, pathogens intrude easily, that leads to vaginitis. Young girls and postmenopausal women are more liable to infection than pubertal and child-bearing period women, in that they lack estrogen, their epithelium of the vagina is very thin, intracellular glycogen decreases, the vagina ph value is around 7, the resistance of the vagina is weak.

Levels:
- High: inflammation and discharge occurs
- Low: The vagina is healthy and normal

Pelvic Inflammatory Disease coefficient:

The pelvic inflammatory disease (PID) occurs around the feminine pelvic cavity. The reproductive organ which is the womb contracts the pelvic cavity peritoneum inflammation genitals' a bacterium retro-infection, which arrives at the pelvic cavity through the womb oviduct.

The female reproductive system has the natural defense function, in normal conditions, it can resist bacterium's invasion. The female natural defense function is destroyed. From this causes scar adhesion which causes pelvic cavity hyperemia. Chronic inflammation may cause the underbelly to fall and it will ache and the waist, shin bone will get sore. This soreness will intensify during sexual intercourse around the menstruation time.

Appendagitis coefficient:

This is an inflammation of the uterine appendages (adnexa).

Cervicitis coefficient:

Cervicitis in a woman of child-bearing age is a common disease, it occurs as acute and chronic. There are two kinds of acute cervicitises. They often exist with the acute womb intimitis or the acute vaginitis. But the main issue of chronic cervicitis is that the leucorrhea (whitish, yellowish vaginal discharge) sticks to the thick purulent mucilage. In normal cases if the vaginal discharge has the consistency of egg whites, means that you are making a lot of estrogen. It often occurs in the middle between your cycles and is a sign of ovulating (your body is releasing an egg) and you are fertile (able to become pregnant).

Levels:
- High: When it is reading high, one of the possible causes can be sexually transmitted infections. Most often, the bacterial and viral infections that cause cervicitis are transmitted by sexual contact. Cervicitis can result from common sexually transmitted infections (STIs), including gonorrhea, chlamydia, trichomoniasis and genital herpes. Also there can be bleeding between menstrual periods, pain with intercourse or during a cervical exam.
- Solution: Doctors commonly prescribe antibiotics as a treatment for cervicitis. These drugs help to clear the infection, which helps to treat symptoms. If cervicitis is caused by an STI, the doctor can advise on the best course of treatments. STIS are often treatable with antibiotics.

Ovarian Cyst Coefficient:

The ovarian cysts are generalized on the different kinds of tumor on the ovaries, each kind are different due to age, kind of sickness, but most are ovarian cysts in 20-50 year old females. Some of the symptoms are where the lower abdomen aches. Also in the lower abdomen clinical leucorrhea increases. The leucorrhea color is yellow and has an unusual smell, menstruation is abnormal and moreover in the usual lower abdomen area, there usually is one solid tumour. However sometimes there is an indolence tumour. Furthermore during sexual intercourse person will experience pain. The cyst will affect the hormone production as well. Also there is a possibility where the vagina can have an anomalous hemorrhage and the tumour increases in size.

An ovarian cyst is a kind of a generalized tumor that is seen in 20-50 year old females. Also an increase in abdominal pain and leucorrhea (whitish, yellowish vaginal discharge) may occur with an unusual smell during menstruation. The solid cyst usually occurs in the lower abdominal area.

Levels:
- High: Severe symptoms can be pelvic pain, dull lower back ache and thighs, problems emptying the bladder and bowels completely, pain during intercourse, breast tenderness, pain during period and unusual vaginal bleeding.
- Low: Some of the symptoms are painful sexual intercourse, abdominal swelling or feeling of fullness or pressure and some mild abdominal ache.

Breast

HYPERPLASIA OF MAMMARY GLANDS COEFFICIENT

This refers to the abnormal increase of the cells that make up the epithelial and fibrous tissue of the mammary glands of the breasts; degenerative change of breast tissue duct, lobule structure and progressive growth of connective tissue. The main reason for this overgrowth is endocrine dyscrasia,
Levels:
- High: When there is an overgrowth of the cells that line the ducts or the milk glands (lobules) inside the breast.

ACUTE MASTITIS COEFFICIENT

It is the Inflammation of the mammary gland of the female breast. It can be caused by chemical agents but usually is from bacterial infection of some kind. This can be diagnosed medically from a bacteriological examination or by indirect tests of the cell count of the milk.

Levels:
- High: Symptoms can vary from pain, heat and swelling of the affected quarter or half of the gland. Also abnormal characteristics of the milk such as clots or flakes and wateriness of the liquid phase may occur.
- Low: a mild case may get better without any medical treatment. If you notice a tender swollen area in your breast when you're breast-feeding, it may be a blocked milk duct or mastitis developing

CHRONIC MASTITIS COEFFICIENT

This occurs in women who are not breastfeeding. In postmenopausal women, breast infections may be associated with chronic inflammation of the ducts below the nipple. Hormonal changes in the body can cause the milk ducts to become clogged with dead skin cells and debris. These clogged ducts make the breast more open to bacterial infection. The Infection can come back after treatment with antibiotics.

ENDOCRINE DYSCRASIA COEFFICIENT

This is when the endocrine system of glands such as the thyroid gland, pituitary, etc. and hormones go out of balance in females, causing such things as skin deterioration, increased emotional anger, gynecological diseases such as dysmenorrheal and breast cancer.

FIBROADENOMA OF BREAST COEFFICIENT

This is a benign (non-cancerous) tumor that is found in the breast of woman usually under the age of 30. African American women tend to develop this kind of tumor more. It is made up of mainly breast tissue and connective (stroma) tissue. They also do not turn into cancer. Although the main cause of this is unknown, hormones such as estrogen may have a part in the growth and development of this tumor. Taking birth control before the age of 20 also has been linked to higher risk of developing this tumor. They will grow more during pregnancy and they often shrink during menopause. They also can shrink on their own at their own time.

Endocrine System

THYROID SECRETION INDEX

Definition: Thyroid is an important organ in the endocrine system. Endocrine system plays a role in regulating other body organs. Thyroid is the largest endocrine gland, when stimulated by your nervous system; it has a physiological effect after being sent to the corresponding organ in the body.

PARATHYROID HORMONE SECRETION INDEX

Definition: The parathyroid hormone affects the metabolism of calcium and phosphorous, mobilizing calcium from the bones to increase calcium concentration in blood. It also helps in the re-absorption of calcium, thereby, maintaining the stability of calcium.
Levels:
- If parathyroid secretion levels are low, calcium concentration is decreased.
- If parathyroid secretion levels are high, excessive absorption may lead to bone fractures.

ADRENAL GLAND INDEX

Definition: The adrenal glands produce a wide variety of hormones and help regulate blood pressure and electrolyte balance in the body. These glands can often be overworked from stress and overuse of stimulants such as coffee, sugar and refined foods.

Levels:
- High: The increased release of these stress hormones can help increase blood pressure, heart rate, elevate blood glucose, and mobilize reserve substances in the body to prepare for any extreme struggle in the external environment.
- Low: Too little stimulation of the adrenal gland can lead to severe abdominal pains,
- vomiting, depression, muscle weakness, fatigue, low blood pressure, weight loss, kidney failure, and changes in mood and personality.

PITUITARY SECRETION INDEX

Definition: The Pituitary Secretion Index plays an important role on metabolism, growth, development and reproduction, by telling other membranes of the endocrine system to work harder or slow down.

Levels:
- High: An over-reactive pituitary gland can lead to weight loss, rapid or irregular heart-beats, fragile bones, excessive facial hair in women, tendency to bruise easily, change of facial structure and a disruption of normal reproductive functions in men and women. It is most commonly caused by noncancerous tumors. This causes the gland to secrete too much of certain kinds of hormones related to growth, reproduction, and metabolism, among other things. Therefore, some people experience gigantism where they continue to grow abnormally.
- Low: Under-reactive pituitary glands can be asymptomatic or can cause symptoms such as low blood pressure, weight loss, depression, nausea, vomiting, constipation, weight gain, thirst, urination, irregular menstrual periods for women, lack of interest in sexual activity, erectile dysfunction. Trauma may cause your pituitary gland to stop producing enough of one or more of its hormones. For example, if you had brain surgery, a brain infection, or a head injury, may affect your pituitary gland. Certain tumors can also affect the function of this gland.

PINEAL SECRETION INDEX

Definition: The pineal gland regulates wake and sleep hormones. Pineal Gland secretion is affected by light and darkness. Its cyclical secretion is closely related to the sexual cycle of humans, as well as to the menstrual cycle of women.

Levels:
- High: During darkness, the secretion will be at its highest.
- Low: During periods of light, secretion will be inhibited

THYMUS GLAND SECRETION INDEX

Definition: The Thymus Gland secretes a hormone called thymosin, which stimulates the development of disease fighting cells, known as T-cells. After puberty, it slowly begins to de-grade; however, the thymus produces all the T-cells by the time puberty reaches.

Levels:
- High: Increase in thymosin may produce a disease called myasthenia gravis, which can cause sudden weakness in your voluntary muscle control.
- Low: Underactive thymus may cause weak immune system and immune deficiency diseases due to the lack of disease fighting cells (i.e. T cells). Malnutrition and protein deficiency can lead to slow or limited growth of the thymus, which will impair the normal function of T-cells.

GLAND SECRETION INDEX

Definition: Gland Secretion Index refers to testis in males and ovaries in women.
Testis secretes the male hormone testosterone and male reproductive cells known as sperm. The function of testosterone is to promote growth. Abnormal growth in the testis can lead to testicular cancer causing symptoms such as swelling so that the testicle is larger than usual or pain or dull ache in the scrotum can also occur.
Ovaries secrete follicle stimulating hormone, progesterone, relaxin and male hormones. They function to enlarge the breast and sexual female characteristics. It also helps proliferate the uterus and maintain the body water, sodium, calcium and lower blood sugar. Relaxin helps to promote loose ligaments in the cervix to help in childbirth. It also enables women to have masculine sexual characteristics. Ovaries also produce the female reproductive cells known as eggs.

Levels:
- Low: When the development of the gonads, sexual characteristics is not happening completely
- protein synthesis is weak in the body. There is reduced sperm production which can lead to infertility in males.
- Ovaries can be underworked in females which are caused by genetic factors or
- autoimmune disorders. Women can develop symptoms of menopause such as hot flashes, mood swings, night sweats, or irregular periods.
- High: Over working of the ovaries in women can cause mild to moderate abdominal pain,
- production of small amounts of urine, and get low protein levels in the blood.
- Abnormally high testosterone levels can be caused by: Tumors: Adrenal and testicular tumors may cause abnormally high testosterone. Anabolic steroid abuse: Sometimes used by athletes and bodybuilders to build more muscle mass or increase athletic performance. Some athletes take Clomid illegally to boost performance.
- Men with high testosterone can experience a variety of troubling symptoms and possible health consequences. Excess testosterone can lead to more aggressive and irritable behaviour

- More acne and oily skin, even worse sleep apnea (if you already have it), and an increase in muscle mass.

Immune System

LYMPH NODE INDEX

Definition: The lymph Node produces lymphocytes (disease-fighting cells) which kill bacteria that enter your body. Lymph nodes can get overworked due to viruses, toxic products of metabolism, certain chemicals, foreign matter, and degeneration of tissue components. Thus, enlarged lymph nodes are a warning device for the person.

Levels:
- High: General swelling of lymph nodes throughout your body. When this occurs, it may indicate an infection, such as HIV or mononucleosis, or an immune system disorder, such as lupus or rheumatoid arthritis. Hard, fixed, rapidly growing nodes, indicating a possible cancer or lymphoma.
- Low: In this case, the lymph node is not swelling, no infection, no disease

TONSIL IMMUNE INDEX

Definition: Tonsils are the first line of defense against ingested or inhaled pathogens. They have specialized cells (antigens) that provoke an immune response by producing antibodies. One of the antibodies produced is called Immunoglobulin A (IgA), which inhibit bacterial adhesion to the respiratory mucosa, and inhibit bacterial growth to neutralize and inhibit the spreading of viruses. Infections may cause the tonsils to become red and painful which is known as tonsillitis. Enlargement of the tonsils is known as tonsil hypertrophy, which cause symptoms such as snoring, bad breath, mouth breathing, decreased appetite, and long standing fatigue.

Levels:
- High: When the tonsil's immune system is high the white blood cells which reside in them kill off the germs entering the body through the throat and palate.

- Low: When the tonsil's immune system is low you can end up with tonsillitis, which can obstruct the airway and cause snoring, nasal congestion, and mouth breathing. Sometimes chronic tonsillitis can lead to more severe conditions like sleep apnea, heart and lung problems.

Solution: To keep tonsils healthy, here are some health tips:
1. Gargle with salt water. Gargling can ease inflammation and reduce discomfort.
2. Practice good oral hygiene. ...
3. Stop smoking immediately. ...
4. Use mouthwash.

BONE MARROW INDEX

Definition: Bone Marrow is where blood cells are produced. Red bone marrow manufactures red blood cells, white blood cells and platelets. Platelets help in haemostasis (arresting of bleeding), white blood cells (leukocytes) kill and suppress a variety of pathogens, including bacteria and viruses. Some of the leukocytes produce antibodies. Therefore, the bone marrow is both a blood-forming and an immune-based organ. Bone Marrow failure is mainly caused by aplastic anemia (body stops producing red cells) which has symptoms such as fatigue, shortness of breath, rapid or irregular heart rate, pale skin, bruising and bleeding.

Levels:
- Low: When bone marrow count is low most experts believe aplastic anemia occurs because your immune system attacks and kills your stem cells in your bone marrow. This causes you to have low blood counts for all three types of blood cells. Low blood counts result in symptoms such as fatigue, tiredness, bleeding, bruising and a higher risk of infection.
- High: A reticulocyte count (retic count) measures the number of reticulocytes in the blood. If the count is too high or too low, it can mean a serious health problem, including anemia and disorders of the bone marrow, liver, and kidneys.

SPLEEN INDEX
Definition: The spleen functions to filter and store blood. Spleen rupture can cause serious bleeding, which is easy to break in the event of a strong external force.

Levels:
- High: Hyper-spleen function can occur due to diseases such as hemolytic anemias (rapid breakdown of red blood cells), and leukemia. When your spleen's overactive, or "hyper," it removes too many blood cells, including healthy ones. Without enough healthy, mature blood cells, your body has a harder time fighting infections and you may become anemic.
- Low: You have an enlarged spleen. In some cases, your spleen can become so large that you may feel pain or fullness in the left upper portion of your chest. You may also have no symptoms, although your doctor can feel an enlarged spleen when checking your ab-do-men.

THYMUS INDEX

Produces lymphocytes and aids in producing immunity. The weight of the thymus shrinks as a person goes from childhood to puberty and from puberty to adulthood. Immunodeficiency can result in the thymus under-functioning.

Levels:
- Low: Removal of the organ in the adult has little effect, but when the thymus is removed in the newborn, T-cells in the blood and lymphoid tissue are depleted, and failure of the immune system causes a gradual, fatal wasting disease," according to Encyclopedia Britannica.
- High: Thymosin is the hormone of the thymus, and enough of it is released to stimulate the development of disease fighting T cells

IMMUNOGLOBULIN INDEX

Definition: Immunoglobulins are antibodies that contribute to immunity in the body. Immunoglobulins can be divided into 5 categories: IgA (mucosal immunity), IgE (allergy and asthma immunity), IgM (appears early in the course of infection), IgG(controls infection of body tissues), IgD (signals specialized cells to become activated so they can take part in defense of the body).

Levels:
If the levels of immunoglobulin are low, it can lead to respiratory problems, sinus and ear infections, and gastrointestinal disorders.
If the levels of immunoglobulin are high, it can lead to enlarged tonsils, immune system dysfunction, enlarged liver, enlarged spleen and anemia.

RESPIRATORY INDEX

The human respiratory system is the main gateway connected with the outside world. Pathogenic microorganisms and harmful substances can lead to inflammatory diseases which can enter into the respiratory tract. Many of the air particles get trapped within the walls of the nasal passages before they can reach the lungs. Mucus, which is produced by specialized cells lining the airway walls, is sticky and traps a great deal of the inhaled dust, pollen, bacteria and viruses.

GASTROINTESTINAL IMMUNE INDEX

GI index is the immunity that includes the full digestive tract from mouth to rectum, all decomposition enzymes, bile, liver barrier and normal flora. It is important that immunity is fully activated in the GI tract because the lumen of the GI tract is outside the body and much of it is heavily populated with potentially pathogenic organisms. The GI immunity can be affected by autoimmune disorders which are conditions that happen when the body's own immune system attacks part of the gastrointestinal tract.

MUCOSA IMMUNE INDEX

Definition: The mucosa immune index provides protection to the person's mucous membranes from invasion of pathogenic microorganisms.

Heavy Metals

LEAD

Definition: Lead is a heavy metal that has no physiological function, so the ideal blood level should be zero. However, due to environmental conditions, the majority of the human body has more or less the presence of lead.

Levels:

High: Lead poisoning can lead to high blood pressure, abdominal, constipation, joint pains, muscle pains, decline in mental functioning, headache, memory loss, reduced sperm count, miscarriage and mood disorders.

CADMIUM

Definition: Cadmium is not an essential element in the human body. It is accumulated in the human body through the air, food and water.

Levels:

Low: Then cadmium absorption can be significantly increased. Intake of zinc can inhibit cadmium absorption. Cadmium content of organs and tissues may vary due to regional differences, environmental pollution and increases with age.

High: It causes respiratory irritation; long-term exposure can cause loss of sense of smell disorders and can cause liver and kidney damage. 60% of cadmium is stored in both the liver and kidney.

ARSENIC

Definition: Arsenic is an essential trace element. It is present in our drinking water and food as the source of arsenic comes from plants, water and air.

Levels:

High: Excessive intake of arsenic may change the way cells communicate, and reduce their ability to function. It can also play a role in the development of diabetes, vascular disease and lung disease.

CHROMIUM

Definition: Chromium is an essential trace element in glucose and lipid metabolism. There are two forms of chromium: hexavalent and trivalent, which is toxic and trivalent, which is beneficial. Chromium in natural foods, are in the trivalent form.

Levels:

High: Hexavalent chromium (produced by industrial processes used in paints, inks, dye sand plastics) targets the respiratory system, kidneys, liver, skin and eyes. This can lead to chronic poisoning of the aforementioned organs.

MERCURY:

Definition: Mercury is a toxic element when inhaled or ingested. Neurological abnormalities can result if mercury is inhaled long-term.

The main acute organ of mercury toxicity is the kidney, followed by the gastrointestinal tract. The main target for chronic toxicity is the brain.

Levels:

High: Mercury poisoning causes inhibition of essential biochemical reactions that take place daily in the body, immune system dysfunctions, and creation of oxygen free-radicals (leading to tissue damage).

ANTIMONY

Definition: Antimony is a silvery white metal which can cause irritation of the eyes, nose, throat and skin upon inhalation. Antimony can be found in the air near industries that process metal, such as coal fired power plants, smelters and refuse incinerators. It can also be found in the natural environment. The general population is exposed to low levels of it through air, drinking water and food.
Levels:
High: High levels of antimony can cause vomiting, headaches, breathing difficulties and severe exposure can even cause death.

THALLIUM

Definition: Thallium is a malleable gray material, which enters the environment through coal burning and smelting. It is a strong nerve poison.
Levels:
High: High levels of thallium can affect kidney and liver function. Inhalation and absorption of thallium through the skin can cause acute poisoning. Prolonged exposure can lead to chronic poisoning.

Vitamins

VITAMIN A

Definition: Vitamin A, also known as retinol, helps your eyes adjust when you come inside from the outdoors and also aids in keeping your skin, mucous membranes and eyes moist. It also has antioxidant properties that aid in neutralizing free radicals in the body that cause cell and tissue damage.

Levels:

- If Vitamin A levels are high, it indicates an overconsumption of Vitamin A which is linked with increased fractures in post-menopausal women. It can possibly cause growth retardation, hair loss, enlarged spleen and liver. Overdose of Vitamin A can also cause birth defects.
- If Vitamin A levels are low, it indicates a deficiency, which is rare. However, Vitamin A deficiency can cause night blindness, eye inflammation, diarrhea and other problems.

VITAMIN B1

Definition: Vitamin B1 is also called Thiamine which is a necessary part of our diet. Thiamine plays a role in carbohydrate metabolism. It also aids in the nervous system and is essential for important body enzymes to function. These body enzymes are involved in processes that provide energy available in the body. Thiamine is necessary for the transmission for certain types of nerve signals between the brain and spinal cord.
Levels:
- If Vitamin B1 levels are high, it generally indicates no concern.
- If Vitamin B1 levels are low, it can indicate depression, poor memory, muscle weakness and stiffness, nerve tingling, tiredness, headache, loss of appetite and nausea.

VITAMIN B2

Definition: Vitamin B2 plays an important role in the body's energy activation and production. It is essential in metabolic activities of the body.

Levels:
- If Vitamin B2 levels are high, it is generally not a concern.
- If Vitamin B2 levels are low, it can indicate B2 deficiency, which can cause symptoms such as excessive sensitivity to light, burning and itching in and around the eyes and loss of clear vision and soreness around the lips, mouth and tongue. Other symptoms can include peeling of the skin, mainly around the nose, or in men around the scrotum.

VITAMIN B3

Definition: Vitamin B3, also called niacin, is essential for conversion of the body's proteins, fats, and carbohydrates into useable energy. Niacin is also used to synthesize starch that can be stored in the body's muscles and liver for later energy use.

Levels:
- If Vitamin B3 levels are high, it is generally not a concern.
- If Vitamin B3 levels are low, it can result in general weakness, muscular weakness and lack of appetite. Digestive problems and skin infections can be associated with niacin deficiency.

VITAMIN B6

Definition: Vitamin B6 is involved with more than 100 enzymatic reactions, and has diverse functions in the human body and comes in a variety of chemical forms. Vitamin B6 was referred to as "antidermatitis factor because skin inflammation (dermatitis) seemed to increase when foods containing vitamin B6 were eliminated from the diet.

Levels:
- If Vitamin B6 levels are high, it can lead to imbalances in the nervous system.
- If Vitamin B6 levels are low, it can indicate a deficiency in Vitamin B6. Symptoms include anemia, fatigue and malaise.

VITAMIN B12

Definition: Vitamin B12 has a variety of forms. However out of all the forms, the only form of B12 that is able to be immediately absorbed and assimilated by the body is the methylcobalamin form.

Levels:
- If Vitamin B12 levels are high, it is generally not a concern.
- If the Vitamin B12 levels are low, it indicates a B12 deficiency. The general symptoms are depression, heart palpitations, fatigue, memory problems, nervousness and numbness in the feet.

VITAMIN C

Definition: Vitamin C helps form collagen which is a fibrous protein in bone, cartilage, tendons, and other connective tissue. Vitamin C aids in providing structure and maintaining body parts such as bones, cartilage, muscle, veins, capillaries and teeth. It also supports the cardiovascular system by facilitating fat metabolism and protecting tissues from free radical damage.

Levels:

Levels:
- If Vitamin C levels are high, it generally indicates the body may not be properly absorbing and assimilating the levels properly. Excessively high levels of Vitamin C can lead to diarrhea.
- If Vitamin C levels are low, it indicates a Vitamin C deficiency, which can lead to scurvy (including bleeding gums and skin discoloration due to ruptured blood vessels); poor wound healing, weak immune function, respiratory infection or other lung related conditions.

VITAMIN D3

Definition: Vitamin D3 aids in the regulation of bone growth, regulation of muscle health, regulation of immune response, regulation of insulin and blood sugar, and regulation of calcium and phosphorous metabolism.

Levels:
- If the Vitamin D3 levels are high, it indicates an elevated level of Vitamin D3 in the body, which can be toxic. Symptoms include loss of appetite, nausea, vomiting, high blood pressure, kidney malfunction, and failure to thrive.
- If the Vitamin D3 levels are low, it indicates Vitamin D3 deficiency. Bone pain, frequent bone fractures and softening of the bones are some of the symptoms.

VITAMIN E

Definition: Vitamin E helps prevent oxidative overload by working together with a group of nutrients that prevent the oxygen molecule from becoming too reactive. The group of nutrients includes Vitamin C, selenium, glutathione and Vitamin B3.

Levels:
- If the Vitamin E levels are high, it indicates excess levels of Vitamin E in the body, which can cause symptoms such as intestinal cramps, fatigue, double vision and muscle weakness.
- If the Vitamin E levels are low, it indicates low levels of Vitamin E which can cause problems such as pancreatic disease, gallbladder disease, liver disease and celiac disease.

VITAMIN K

Definition: Vitamin K is an important vitamin in promoting normal blood coagulation and bone growth. Vitamin K is the essential substance in the synthesis of blood clotting proteins in the liver.

Levels:
- If Vitamin K levels are high, it is generally not a concern.
- If Vitamin K levels are low, it indicates a Vitamin K deficiency. People deficient in Vitamin K are more likely to have symptoms related to problematic blood clotting or bleeding. Symptoms include heavy menstrual bleeding, gum bleeding, bleeding in the digestive tract, nose bleeding, easy bruising, blood in urine, anemia, hemorrhage and prolonged clotting times. Other secondary symptoms as a result of Vitamin K deficiency involves bone problems, which includes loss of bone, osteoporosis, fractures, excess deposit of calcium in soft tissues which can harden the arteries and cause problems in the function of heart valves.

Amino Acids

LYSINE

Definition: Lysine is an amino acid that enhances the development of the brain. It helps in preventing cell degradation and enhances fat metabolism. It regulates the pineal gland, corpus luteum, ovary and the lactiferous glands.

Levels:
- Lack of lysine may cause low gastric secretion, which will lead to anorexia and nutritional anemia, which results in central nervous system disruption and dysplasia.
- If Lysine levels are high, it is generally not a concern.

TRYPTOPHAN

Definition: Tryptophan promotes the production of gastric and pancreatic juices. It also aids in improving the sleep duration of an individual.

Levels:
- If Tryptophan levels are high, it can cause a disease known as Hartnup disease, which is a disorder of amino acid transport in the kidneys and intestine. Symptoms include physical stress, fever, rashes when exposed to the sun, anxiety, rapid mood changes, delusions and hallucinations.
- If Tryptophan levels are low, it can lead to anxiety, depression, withdrawal from social life, low appetite, difficulty sleeping, hopelessness and low self-image. In severe cases, low tryptophan levels can cause dementia.

PHENYLALANINE

Definition: Phenylalanine helps to promote the production of gastric juice and pancreatic juice. It is one of the essential amino acids in the human body, which is ingested through food intake.

Levels:
- If Phenylalanine levels are low, it indicates phenylalanine deficiency, which can cause symptoms such as confusion, decreased alertness, depression, sluggish metabolism, lack of energy, faulty memory and reduced appetite. An inability to metabolize phenylalanine is a rare genetic disorder that leads to mental retardation in newborns if not treated.
- If Phenylalanine levels are high, IQ deficits, vomiting and more pronounced developmental abnormalities can result.

METHIONINE

Definition: Methionine is an essential amino acid that assists in metabolic function, breaks down fat and is the primary source of sulphur in the body. It can protect liver cells from destruction.

Levels:
- If Methionine levels are low, it can trigger symptoms like elevated cholesterol levels and liver damage.
- If Methionine levels are high, it can increase the risk for dementia.

![Vital Health logo] *Helping people rebuild from the inside out.*

THREONINE

Definition: Threonine is an essential amino acid that helps to maintain the proper protein balance in the body.

Levels:
If Threonine levels are too high in babies can increase brain glycine levels which will affect the neurotransmitter balance in the brain which can affect brain development.
If Threonine levels are low, it can cause depression or excessive nervousness. Other symptoms can include digestive problems, and in severe cases, liver failure.

ISOLEUCINE

Definition: Isoleucine participates in the regulation and metabolism of the thymus, spleen and pituitary gland. It is also an essential amino acid.

Levels:
If Isoleucine levels are High for a long time, studies have shown that it contributes to the development of triglyceride levels increasing in the body.
If Isoleucine levels are low, symptoms such as confusion, irritability, fatigue, depression, dizziness and headaches can result.

LEUCINE

Definition: Leucine is an essential amino acid that increases muscle mass and helps muscles recover after exercise. It also regulates blood sugar and supplies the body with energy.
Levels:
- If Leucine levels are high, ammonia can accumulate in the body. Excess ammonia circulating in the bloodstream may cause tissue damage and organ failure. This is a rare case, due to the fact that it requires an extreme high level of leucine in the blood.
- If Leucine levels are low, it can indicate leucine deficiency. Symptoms include headaches, fatigue, dizziness, depression, confusion and irritability.

VALINE

Definition: Valine is an amino acid that prevents the breakdown of muscle, because it supplies muscles with extra glucose responsible for the production of energy during physical activity.

Levels:
- High valine levels cause the "failure to thrive" condition in infants and small children in which they have physical and mental retardation. Valine excess can be seen in people with

hypoglycemia (low blood sugar level), and with visual and tactile hallucinations.
- If Valine levels are low, it can lead to Valine deficiency. The inability to metabolize, leucine, isoleucine and valine cause Maple Syrup disease. It is named Maple Syrup disease because the urine from these affected people smells like maple syrup. Valine deficiencies can be seen in people when they are in a state of hunger, obesity, neurological deficit and with elevated insulin levels.

HISTIDINE

Definition: Histidine aids in providing protection to neural cells, detoxification of heavy metals, and manufacturing of white and red blood cells, aiding in proper digestion, promoting proper sexual function and assisting with immunity.

Levels:
- If Histidine levels are high, it can lead to stress and mental disorders such as anxiety. It can also contribute to the start of schizophrenia.
- If Histidine levels are low, it can lead to rheumatoid arthritis, and can be linked with nerve deafness.

ARGININE

Definition: Arginine is involved in many metabolic processes, and important in the treatment of heart diseases and high blood pressure. Arginine improves the circulation and strengthens the immune system.14

Levels:
- If Arginine levels are low, it can lead to hypertension, low sperm count, loss of hair, skin rash, constipation, arterioschlerosis, poor wound healing, fatty liver, alkalosis and diminished insulin production.
- If Arginine levels are high, it can delay growth in children, cause developmental delays, vomiting, poor appetite, breathing trouble, small head size, sleeping longer than normal, and tight, rigid muscles. The aforementioned signs can be seen from infancy to childhood.

Allergen

BACTERIAL ALLERGY
Definition: There are a variety of bacteria in the air that can cause allergies. Drinking plenty of water, exercise and rest are some useful techniques to improve one's immunity.

ANTIBIOTICS
Definition: Antibiotics are medicines that kill or inhibit bacterial growth. Although antibiotics can usually help the immune system fight off those infections, overuse of antibiotics is leading to the growing number of bacterial infections that are becoming resistant to antimicrobial drugs.

HETEROLOGOUS SERUM
Definition: The heterologous system is serum (portion of blood) that is obtained from an animal belonging to a species different from the recipient. This will trigger the body to produce antibodies which can target specific infections/diseases.

CAIN MIXTURE
Definition: Cain mixture is found in many anesthetics which cause damage to specialized cells (mast cells), causing redness of the skin, edema and whealing (swelling on skin).

EPOXY
Definition: This is present in adhesives, surface coatings and paints which cause damage to specialized cells (mast cells), causing redness of the skin, edema and whealing (swelling on skin).

QUINOLINE MIX
Definition: Quinoline mix is present in adhesives, surface coatings and paints which cause damage to specialized cells (mast cells), causing redness of the skin, edema and whealing (swelling on skin).

MICROBIAL INFECTIONS
Definition: Microbial infections are one of the most important influences leading to infection by microorganisms (microbes). In humans, 50% of infections are caused by a virus.

IONIZING RADIATION
Definition: Ionizing radiation is a form of radiation that strips electrons from atoms, leaving the nuclei unstable. At high enough doses, upon exposure, ionizing radiation can cause damage to molecules such as DNA. Damage to DNA and other important cellular components can result in cell damage or death. This can lead to health effects like cancer risk, skin damage, blood disorders, fertility damage and pathological changes to the nervous system, blood forming organs and the digestive system.

POTASSIUM DICHROMATE
Definition: Potassium dichromate is present in cement and a variety of chemicals which cause damage to specialized cells (mast cells), causing redness of the skin, edema and whealing (swelling on skin).

KABA MIXTURE
Definition: Kaba mixture exists in a variety of local anesthetics which cause damage to specialized cells (mast cells), causing redness of the skin, edema and whealing (swelling on skin).

ANIMAL HAIR
Definition: Animal hair may contain bacteria, mites and other allergens.

PAINT
Definition: Paints produce vapours that not only create chemical odours in the air, but also an allergic reaction in many people (i.e. coughing, runny nose, sore throat and congestion).

UV
Definition: UV can cause allergies due to sun's ultraviolet rays which penetrate the skin. The allergic areas of the person's body can become red and can burn due to the radiation. UV can also lead to free radicals in the body, causing wrinkling, cell damage, pigmentation, immune system damage which can lead to further allergic reactions.

FORMALDEHYDE
Definition: Formaldehyde exists in a variety of building materials and plastics industries, which cause damage to specialized cells (mast cells), causing redness of the skin, edema and whealing.

LANOLIN ALCOHOL

Definition: Lanolin Alcohol exists in a variety of ointments, creams, skin care products and soap, which cause damage to specialized cells (mast cells), causing redness of the skin, edema and whealing (swelling on skin).

CHLORIDE

Definition: Chloride exists in the gold-plated items and artificial jewelry, which cause damage to specialized cells (mast cells), causing redness of the skin, edema and whealing.

Eye

ORBICULARIS OCULI MUSCLE (EYE INDEX)

Definition: Orbicularis Oculi muscle is the muscle in the face that closes the eyelids. The loss of this function may result in the inability to close the eye.

COLLAGEN WRINKLE EYE

Definition: Collagen is a protein that maintains the structure, smoothness and elasticity of the skin. As a person ages, collagen naturally decreases. The decrease in collagen can lead to wrinkles and baggy eyes.

SKIN PIGMENTATION

Definition: Pigmentation of the iris (circular structure of the eye) varies from light brown to black, depending on the melanin (natural body pigment) concentration of the iris. Hy-per-pigmentation can be seen in African, Mediterranean and Asian ethnicities. Hy-per-pigmentation can cause diseases such as Addison's disease (adrenal insufficiency) and Cushings disease (increase in secretion of ACTH, a hormone produced in response to bio-logical stress).

LYMPHATIC OBSTRUCTION

Definition: The lymphatics in the eye are numerous and extensive. Lymphatic system is part of the circulatory system, which acts as an accessory route to help return excess blood. It also aids in the defense of the immune system. Lymphatic vessels in the eye can become obstructed, which cause the iris to project against the cornea, leading to glaucoma.

RELAXATION UNDER THE VERTICAL

Definition: Relaxation under the vertical is due to sagging between the fiber cells which can lead to cell degradation over time, in which the skin loses its elasticity and causes the skin to become loose.

EDEMA

Definition: Edema is where excess fluid is trapped in the body tissues. If blood vessels leak fluid into the surrounding tissue, that area will start to swell. Edema in the eyes is known as macular edema.

EYE CELL ACTIVITY

Definition: Cell activity is the physiological state and function of cells in the eye. The activity (i.e. metabolism) will decrease as the temperature decreases which can lead to death. High temperatures can also lead to cell death.

VISUAL FATIGUE

Definition: Eye fatigue is caused due to close-form work, computer work, or insufficient lighting. Usual symptoms are: blurred visions, unable to write and read, dry eyes and dizziness.

Obesity

TOLERANCE FUNCTION

Definition: Tolerance function is the ability for your body to metabolize glucose and clear it away from the blood.

Levels:
High values of tolerance indicate metabolic conditions which result in higher than normal blood glucose levels, resulting in pre-diabetes.

LIPID METABOLISM

Definition: Lipid metabolism refers to the degradation and breakdown of lipids.

HIGH INSULIN

Definition: High insulin has a significant role in promoting fat accumulation. Insulin can be used as an indicator of the overall fat content and monitoring of obesity factor. Blood insulin concentration and total fat content have positive correlations.

Bone Growth Index

BONE ALKALINE PHOSPHATASE

Definition: Bone alkaline phosphatase is secreted by the bone, which is a great indicator of bone metabolism. It is found on the surface of bone-forming cells known as osteoblasts. Normal bone is constantly going through a phase of bone formation balanced by bone degradation. Bone alkaline phosphatase is a reflection of the synthetic activity (formation) of bone.. Levels:
High: If the process becomes unbalanced, the rate of degradation exceeds the rate of formation which leads to osteoporosis

OSTEOCALCIN

Definition: Osteocalcin is a protein found in bone which is secreted by osteoblasts. It is used as a marker for bone function.).
Levels:
High: High levels of blood osteocalcin are correlated with treatment with drugs during

osteoporosis (i.e. where bone degradation exceeds the rate of bone formation

STATUS OF LONG BONE HEALING

Definition: Long bone is located mainly in the limbs. It can be divided into one backbone and two ends. Long bones, especially the femur and tibia are subjected to most of the body's daily activities and are crucial for skeletal mobility.

SHORT BONE CARTILAGE HEALING SITUATION

Definition: Short bone cartilage is located in the wrist, foot and the latter part of the spine. Short bone can withstand great pressure, often with multiple tissue surfaces (i.e. articular surface).

EPIPHYSEAL LINE

Definition: The epiphyseal line is a cartilage at each end of the long bone (bones that are longer than they are wide). In adults who have stopped growing, the plate is replaced by an epiphyseal line.

Coenzymes

NICOTINAMIDE

Definition: Nicotinamide is an essential body enzyme which activates a variety of enzyme systems, and promotes nucleic acid, protein and carbohydrate synthesis, regulates material transport in the body and improves one's metabolism.
Levels:
Low levels of nicotinamide are due to vitamin B3 deficiency (found in many foods such as fish, eggs, meat, green vegetables).

BIOTIN

Definition: Biotin is the material necessary for the synthesis of vitamin C, which is essential to normal metabolism of fat and protein substances. It is necessary for the body's natural growth and to maintain normal body function.

Levels:

Low: Biotin deficiency can be associated with excess egg consumption, taking an-ti-bacterial medicines and chronic dieting. Biotin deficiency, however, is very rare as the body recycles much of its biotin.

PANTOTHENIC ACID

Definition: Pantothenic acid helps in the manufacture of energy in the body and can control fat metabolism. It helps in anti-stress hormones (steroids) secretion.

Levels:

Low levels of pantothenic acid is due to vitamin B5 deficiency (meat, legumes, cereal grains, eggs and milk)

FOLIC ACID

Definition: Folic Acid is the necessary material of the body's use of sugars and amino acids and is also the necessary material for body cell growth and reproduction.

Levels:

Low: Low folic acid can lead to anemia (i.e. low hemoglobin levels) and low defense fighting cells (i.e. white blood cells). It can also lead to physical weakness, irritability, loss of ap-petite, and psychiatric symptoms.

COENZYME Q10

Definition: Coenzyme Q10 (found in fish, beef, poultry, nuts, seeds, oils, fruits/vegetables) is indispensable to human life. It is one of the important elements that can activate the body's cells and energy nutrients, improve immunity, enhance anti-oxidation, anti-aging, and enhance the vitality of human body function.

Levels:

Low: Low Levels of Coenzyme Q10 is due to low dietary intake.

GLUTATHIONE

Definition: Glutathione helps the body maintain a normal immune system function. It is an important antioxidant in the body and can rid the body of free radicals and can also clean and purify the human body.

Levels:

Low levels of glutathione are associated with alcoholism, Alzheimer's, cigarette smoking, Parkinson's, and chronic fatigue syndrome.

Sperm and Semen

SEMEN VOLUME
Definition: Semen volume generally decreases as males age. Younger men tend to have high ejaculation volumes. Men with high abdominal fat get an increase in estrogen which can reduce the ejaculatory volume.

LIQUEFYING TIME
Definition: Semen is a thick, viscous fluid. Liquefying time is the measure of time it takes for the semen to liquefy. The liquefying time is usually 20-30 minutes following ejaculation. Prolonged liquefaction time can be due to disorders of accessory gland function.

NUMBER OF SPERMS
Definition: Also known as the total sperm count (normal range is 20-120 million sperm per milliliter of semen). Low sperm count can be due to an obstruction in the ejaculation tract, hormonal insufficiency, testicular injuries, or genetic abnormalities.

SPERM MOTILITY RATE
Definition: The ability of the sperm to swim or be motile. If the sperm motility is low, then it will not make it past the vaginal canal to fertilize the egg. Low sperm motility can be due to stress, heat, lack of vitamins and minerals, heavy metals, excessive sex, smoking, alcohol and genetics.

Pulse of Heart and Brain

CARDIAC STROKE VOLUME
Definition: Cardiac Stroke Volume is the amount of blood pumped by the left ventricle of the

heart during one contraction. However, the heart does not pump all the blood out of the ventricle. Approximately two-thirds of the blood in the ventricle is put out with each beat. Stroke volume is an important factor of cardiac output, which is the product of stroke volume and heart rate. The evaluation of the cardiac output is important in determining the work that the heart is performing with respect to the rest of the cardiovascular system.

Levels:
- If the Cardiac Stroke Volume readings are high, then the heart is working too hard and can lead to heart damage and possibly stroke.
- If the Cardiac Stroke Volume readings are low, then the body is not being properly supplied with blood (heart failure), which can and will lead to life threatening problems if left un-checked.

STROKE INDEX

Definition: Stroke Index is the Stroke Volume divided by the body surface area.

HEART PERIPHERAL RESISTANCE

Definition: The peripheral resistance is the total resistance opposing blood flow when the cardiovascular system carries oxygenated blood away from the heart to the body, and returns deoxygenated blood back to the heart.
Exercising will result in an increased flow to tissues and an increase venous flow back to the heart.
Levels:
Low: Decrease in total peripheral resistance can be due to drugs like cocaine, renal diseases, cortisol levels, and increased intracranial pressure.

BLOOD VESSEL ELASTICITY

Definition: Arteries expand to accept the blood being forced into them from the heart, and then squeeze this blood into the veins upon relaxation of the heart. Arteries have the property of elasticity (i.e. they can expand to when blood flows through them), and then contract and squeeze back to their original size upon release of pressure. A balloon is a good analogy: when you blow into the balloon, it inflates to hold the air. When you release the opening, the balloon squeezes the air back out. It is the elasticity of the arteries that maintains the pressure on the blood when the heart relaxes, and keeps it flowing forward.

Levels:
High blood vessel elasticity readings indicates that the vessels have become less elastic which can lead to a risk for strokes, heart attacks, heart failure and renal failure.
Low blood vessel elasticity readings indicates that the vessels have become weak and can cause light-headedness, dizziness, weakness, fainting and in extreme cases shock.

PULSE WAVE COEFFICIENT K:

Definition: Pulse-wave velocity (PWV) is a measurement of arterial stiffness that is an independent predictor of cardiovascular risk. It can be measured simply and noninvasively by measuring the carotid and femoral pulse pressures and the time delay between the two or by other methods relying on pulse-wave analysis.

High: can mean a stiffer artery, hence higher risk of high blood pressure and heart disease

CEREBROVASCULAR BLOOD OXYGEN SATURATION/VOLUME

Definition: The average cerebral blood flow in humans is approximately 55 ml per 100 g of brain tissue per minute. Almost all oxygen consumed by the brain is utilized for the oxidation of carbohydrates.

Low tissue levels of oxygen in the brain can be caused by decreased blood flow, or with adequate blood flow with low levels of blood oxygen. Comas and convulsions are good examples of how blood oxygen saturation decreases.

CEREBROVASCULAR BLOOD OXYGEN PRESSURE

Definition: Cerebrovascular Blood Oxygen Pressure is the net pressure causing cerebral blood flow to the brain.
Levels:
- If the Cerebrovascular Blood Oxygen Pressure levels are low, it could cause tissue to become ischemic (having inadequate blood flow) which can be due to blood clots and trauma.
- If the Cerebrovascular Blood Oxygen Pressure levels are high, it can raise the intracranial pressure (i.e. the pressure inside the skull, brain tissue and cerebrospinal fluid). This can further lead to altered level of consciousness, vomiting without nausea, back pain or papilledema (increased cranial pressure causing swelling of optic nerve in eye).

Blood Lipids

TOTAL CHOLESTEROL
Definition: Total cholesterol is a measure of the total amount of cholesterol in your blood, including low density lipoprotein (LDL) cholesterol and high density lipoprotein (HDL) cholesterol. LDL (i.e. bad cholesterol) – the main source of cholesterol buildup and blockage in the arteries. HDL (good cholesterol) – HDL removes cholesterol from the arteries Triglycerides – a form of fat in your blood that can increase risks for heart disease. Saturated fat and cholesterol in food can increase blood cholesterol levels. Being overweight is a risk for heart disease and can also increase cholesterol. Physical activity can help lower LDL (bad) cholesterol and increase HDL (good) cholesterol levels. As women and men age, cholesterol levels tend to rise. After the age of menopause, women's LDL levels tend to increase. Genes contribute partially to how much cholesterol your body makes.

NEUTRAL FAT
Definition: Neutral Fats are uncharged fatty acids with glycerol. They cover our torso and legs to provide insulation to keep the body warm and keep body fuel reserves.

CIRCULATING IMMUNE COMPLEX
Definition: CIC is an immune complex containing an antigen (a protein particle provoking an immune response) and an antibody (produced in response to an antigenic stimulus). It is detectable in a variety of disorders such as rheumatology, autoimmune, allergic diseases, viral, bacterial infections and malignancies.

COLLAGEN ANALYSIS (LOSS OF)

EYE: dry eyes, fatigue, spontaneous tears, poor corneal transparency and lens opacity

TOOTH: susceptibility to tooth decay and loss, gum disease, and calcium loss

HAIR AND SKIN: dryness, breaking, hair loss, increased dandruff, increased wrinkles, loose skin, chin and eyes drooping.

ENDOCRINE SYSTEM: menstrual disorders, breast cancer, dysplasia, early entry into menopause, breast sagging and premature ejaculation.

CIRCULATORY SYSTEM: affects stability of blood pressure, high blood cholesterol, fatty liver, susceptibility to cardiovascular and cerebrovascular diseases, memory loss, dizziness, forgetfulness and insomnia.

DIGESTIVE SYSTEM: decreases cardiac pumping, increases waist and abdomen, flatulence, diabetes, weak hematopoietic (blood cell production) function and anemia.

IMMUNE SYSTEM: slow lymphatic circulation leading to decreased immunity, muscle pain and easy infection of epidemic diseases.

MOTION SYSTEM: joint pain, stiffness, poor metabolism, muscle atrophy (cell death), bone deformation, rheumatism, cold hands and feet, numbness of limbs, blocked activity, slow bone healing and loss of calcium.

MUSCLE TISSUE: increase in fat mass, back pain, shoulder tingling, connective tissue block, indurations (hardening) of cervical muscles, poor muscle contractions, loss of energy, muscle pulling force and decreased muscle tone.

FAT METABOLISM: decrease in metabolism, easy fatigue, prone to diabetes, high blood pressure, resulting in liver and kidney failure.

DETOXIFICATION AND METABOLISM: susceptibility to toxin accumulation, constipation, physical obesity, prone to nephritis, itching skin, pain, body acne, mental decline and skin cancer.

REPRODUCTIVE SYSTEM: shedding of the uterus, urinary incontinence, low immunity, re- productive system, dryness, female infertility, male impotence, hemorrhoids, and pelvic pain.

NERVOUS SYSTEM: memory loss, inability to concentrate, insomnia, anxiety, depression, poor response and nerve pain.

SKELETON: decreased bone density, loss of calcium, bone and joint pain, bone spurs, muscle atrophy, bone cancer, leg paralysis and osteoporosis.

Large Intestine Function

LARGE INTESTINE PERISTALSIS FUNCTION COEFFICIENT

Definition: Peristalsis is the involuntary contraction and relaxation of muscles of the intestine, which create wave like movements that push the digested food forward. The large
intestine has similar segmental motion and peristalsis as the small intestine, but with a much lower frequency.
Levels:
* If the level of intestinal peristalsis is too slow, it can lead to constipation.
* If the levels of intestinal peristalsis are too fast, it is a sign of improper digestion of nutrients in the digestive system. A good rule of thumb is to eat and chew slowly and reduce stress.

COLONIC ABSORPTION COEFFICIENT

Definition: Colonic Absorption is the absorption of water and electrolytes (sodium and chloride ions) back into the body.
Pathological factors such as colitis will reduce the absorption of water and sodium in the large intestine.
If levels are too low, meaning not enough fluid is being absorbed by the colon (Large Intestine) it can be due to some kind of colonic disease which then can lead to the 1.5 L of abnormal fluid, water and electrolytes not being absorbed, hence causing diarrhea.
If levels are too high, meaning too much fluid is being absorbed by the colon which can cause the stool to become dry and hard, hence constipation will occur.
Solution: Slow or delayed bowel movements can be caused by a lack of fiber in your diet. A diet that emphasizes natural, unprocessed fruit and vegetables can kick-start digestion and help make you more regular unless you have IBS, gastroparesis or other chronic gastrointestinal condition.

INTESTINAL BACTERIA COEFFICIENT

Definition: Healthy intestinal bacteria produce by-products that help keep the intestinal lining strong, improve digestion, strengthen the immune system and manufacture essential vitamins for the body.
However, if the ratio of bad to good bacteria is high, the intestinal tract becomes susceptible

to damage. This can cause inflammation which allows undigested food particles, disease causing bacteria and toxins to pass directly into the blood stream. As a result, the body's normal function can be disrupted in many ways. Symptoms include constipation, excess intestinal gas, chronic bad breath and chronic diarrhea.

When the ratio of good bacteria is too low compared to the bad bacteria autoimmune issue start to occur such as thyroid problems, rheumatoid arthritis and type 1 diabetes. Also digestive issues such as irritable bowel syndrome, constipation, diarrhea, heartburn or bloating, sleep issues, skin rashes, allergies and sugar cravings (note. This may come from the proliferation of parasites that feed on the sugar)
Solution: Some of the lifestyle changes that can be made to correct the imbalance in good gut flora are, focus on whole quality organic foods, eat more fiber, increase anti-inflammatory fats, eliminate the foods that feed the bad bacteria, eat and drink more fermented foods, eat food that feed the good bacteria, exercise regularly and get proper sleep.

Thyroid

FREE THYROXINE (FT4)

Definition: Free T4 is the most important biochemical test in determining how the thyroid is functioning.
Levels:
If free T4 is high, then hyperthyroidism is present (symptoms include fatigue or muscle weakness, hand tremors, mood swings, anxiety, skin dryness and trouble sleeping.)
If Free T4 levels are low, then hypothyroidism is present (symptoms include fatigue, weakness, weight gain, hair loss, cold intolerance and rough pale skin).

THYROGLOBULIN

Definition: Thyroglobulin is a protein used to produce the thyroid hormones T3 (triiodo-thyronine) and T4(thyroxine). The thyroglobulin blood test is primarily used as a tumor marker to monitor thyroid cancer and to monitor for recurrence.
Levels:
• Thyroglobulin levels are usually high in people who have thyroid cancer, but your

thyroglobulin level can still be high even without cancer which is known as a benign thyroid condition. High levels of thryoglobulin can also be associated with thyroid inflammation, goiter, or hyperthyroidism.

• Low amounts of thryoglobulin are normal with those who have normal thyroid function. As for a person diagnosed with thyroid cancer, thyroglobilin levels should be low or undetectable after surgical removal of the thyroid or after subsequent radioactive iodine treatments.

ANTI THYROGLOBULIN ANTIBODIES

Definition: Anti-thyroglobulin antibodies are proteins (antibodies) that bind to the protein thyroglobulin.
Levels:
• If anti-thyroglobulin levels are low or normal, it is of no clinical significance.
• If anti-thyroglobulin levels are high, it can be due to graves disease, hypothyroidism, systemic lupus erythematosus, type 1 diabetes and thyroid inflammation(thryoiditis).

TRIIODOTHYRONINE (T3)

Definition: T3 AND T4, are hormones that regulate the body's temperature, metabolism and heart rate.
Levels:
• If T3 levels are high, it might indicate thyroid issues such as, graves' disease, hyper-thyroidism, thyroiditis and goiter.
• If T3 levels are low, it can indicate starvation or hypothyroidism. T3 levels are known to decrease when you are sick.

ADHD GE NEUROTRANSMITTERS

Definition: Glycine Encephalopathy is an autosomal (type of chromosomes placement in the DNA) recessive disorder of the metabolism of glycine. It is characterized by high levels of the amino acid glycine especially in cerebrospinal fluid.
Levels:
High levels of GE neurotransmitters indicate a high amount of glycine in the frontal cortex of the brain. There are several forms of the disease that are caused by this, with varying severity of symptoms and time of onset. The symptoms are exclusively neurological in nature,

Element Of Human Analysis

What do body composition scale readings mean?
The most common readings on a body composition scale are BMI, Body Fat Percentage, Total Body Water, Basal Metabolic Rate, Fat Mass and Fat Free Mass. At Marsden, we've recently updated our body composition scales to deliver a further nine readings - Bone Mineral content, Muscle Mass, Protein Mass, Extracellular Water, Intracellular Water, Skeletal Muscle, Visceral Fat Area level and Health Score.

Body Mass Index (BMI)

BMI is the most common way of determining overall body health and whether a person is underweight or overweight.
To calculate BMI simply divide a person's weight in kilograms by square metres in height. BMI can be calculated on many weighing scales. It is a non-invasive way of assessing body weight - with links drawn between BMI and illness. BMI scales are a popular choice for many users to better understand their body health; however, BMI does not provide an indication of the distribution of body fat.
For more information on healthy BMI, download this helpful BMI infographic poster.

Body Fat Percentage

Body Fat Percentage gives a good indication of body health, but interpreted by itself could give a slightly misleading picture.
The Royal College of Nursing says the healthy target for body fat percentage changes with age. For men aged 20-39, for example, target body fat percentage is 8-20%; after 60 years of age this increases to up to 25%.
Body fat percentage is the proportion of fat mass compared to everything else (bones, muscles and water) and is displayed as a percentage.

Inorganic Substances of the Body

The major inorganic compounds are water (H_2O), bimolecular oxygen (O_2), carbohydrate dioxide (CO_2), and some acids , bases, and salts. The body is composed of 60–75% water.

Helping people rebuild from the inside out.

Total Body Water (TBW)

The Total Body Water measurement shows how hydrated the body is. Water is used in the body for transporting waste, helping organs to function, regulating body temperature and digestion.

The amount of fluid consumption required varies from person to person, and is influenced by climate and the amount of physical activity undertaken. Experts recommend an individual's consumption should be at least two litres of fluid per day.

An average Total Body Water reading for men is 55-60%; for women it is 50-55%.

Basal Metabolic Rate (BMR)

Basal Metabolic Rate is the amount of calories your body needs to function. It is based on the number of calories the body would need if resting for 24 hours. This allows you to calculate an accurate calorie intake target for your body - far more accurate than a generic calculation which might be found online - enabling you to create a diet pro-gramme.

A person with a high BMR burns more calories than a person with a low rate. Around 70% of calories consumed every day are used for your basal metabolism. It fits hand in hand with muscle mass, as the greater the muscle mass, the higher the BMR and the more calories are burned.

Fat Mass and Fat Free Mass (FM/FFM)

Fat Mass is the total mass of the fat in the body and Fat Free Mass is everything else: including bones, muscle and water.

Some body fat is classified 'essential fat' - which the body needs to function, and keep organs warm. Therefore a very low Fat Mass reading can be dangerous.

Calories or energy in the body come from what we eat and drink. Energy is burned from physical activity, but if you consume more than you burn excess calories are stored in fat cells, culminating in excess body fat. Too much body fat can damage long-term health.

You can read more about these readings in this white paper.

Visceral Fat Area level (VFA)

Visceral Fat is the fat which protects vital organs. Ensuring you have a healthy level of visceral fat directly reduces the risk of diseases such as heart disease and high blood pressure.

VFA is used to determine the risk of diabetes, alongside BMI. VFA is shown as a level out of 50, with a score of 41-50 indicating an extremely high risk.

Muscle Mass (MM)

This consists of skeletal muscles, smooth muscles and the water which is contained within them. As muscle mass increases, the rate at which energy is burned increases, accelerating the basal metabolic rate. An increase in muscle mass may increase total body weight, and muscle weighs more than fat. Therefore, it is important to monitor each aspect of the body separately using body composition measurements.

Bone Mineral content (BM)

This tracks the amount of bone mineral found in the body. A higher bone density and strength is indicated by a higher bone mineral content.
Calcium is the largest contributor of bone mineral content. Find out more here.

Protein Mass

Protein Mass tracks the amount of protein in the body. A lack of protein can be linked to an increase in body fats. There is a link between protein mass and muscle mass. As you get older you need more protein due to anabolic resistance, which lowers the body's ability to break down and synthesize protein.

Extracellular Water (ECW)

Water found outside of cells is called Extracellular water - which helps tissue to function well. Nutrients are served to membrane-bound cells via extracellular water, such as sodium, potassium, calcium, chlorides and bicarbohydrates. An increase in extracellular water can cause excess weight and swelling in your limbs. Imbalances may cause symptoms such as decreased mental alertness, nausea and dizziness or result in high blood pressure.. Typically, roughly one third of your body is extra cellular water.

Intracellular Water (ICW)

Water that is located inside your cells is intracellular water - in healthy people it comprises two thirds of the water inside your body. This type of water plays an important role in allowing molecules to be transported to different organelles inside the cell.
Having an increased ICW can signal a positive change in your body composition. When muscle cells become larger, they require more ICW in order to power their cellular functions.

Increased ICW contributing to an increased lean body mass can lead to an improved BMR, increased strength and a better immune system.

Skeletal Muscle (SM)

Skeletal Muscle is one of three major muscle types (alongside cardiac and smooth muscle). It is the most common of the three. These types of muscles are attached to bones by tendons and produce all the movements of body parts in relation to each other.

Metabolic Age (AGEM)

This is worked out by comparing the Basal Metabolic Rate to the average BMR of your age group. If the metabolic age is higher than your actual age, it is a sign that you need to improve your metabolic rate.

Health score

Health score provides an overall score for your body, taking into account height, age, weight and gender information. It is calculated out of 100; the higher the score the better.

David S. Lee   *Helping people rebuild from the inside out.*   **Vital Health**

Endnotes

1. Wardlaw, Gordon M. (4th Edition)(2000). Contemporary Nutrition: Issues And Insights. USA., The McGraw-Hill Companies.

2. Turner, Natasha. (2010). The Hormone Diet: Lose Fat, Gain Strength, Live Younger Longer. Toronto, Canada: Random House of Canada Limited. (pp.14-17)

3. Turner, Natasha. (2010). The Hormone Diet: Lose Fat, Gain Strength, Live Younger Longer. Toronto, Canada: Random House of Canada Limited. (pp.24-28)

4. Turner, Natasha. (2010). The Hormone Diet: Lose Fat, Gain Strength, Live Younger Longer. Toronto, Canada: Random House of Canada Limited. (pp.14-105)

5. http://www.livestrong.com/article/517213-foods-that-stimulate-peristaltic-motion/

6. https://en.wikipedia.org/wiki/Kidney_failure

7. http://drmyhill.co.uk/wiki/hypochlorhydria_-_lack_of_stomach_acid_-_can_cause_lots_of problems

8. http://www.webmd.com/digestive-disorders/digestive-diseases-pancreatitis

9. http://www.niddk.nih.gov/health-information/health-topics/kidney-disease/protein

10. Kapit, Macey, Meisami (2000). The Physiology Coloring Book. San Francisco, CA.: Ben-ja-min/Cummings Science Publishing. (p.58-61)

11. Kapit, Macey, Meisami (2000). The Physiology Coloring Book. San Francisco, CA.: Ben-ja-min/Cummings Science Publishing. (p.51-57)

12. Kapit, Elson (1993). The Anatomy Coloring Book. New York, NY: Harper Collins College Pub-lishers. (p.135-140)

Helping people rebuild from the inside out.

14. Wardlaw, Gordon M. (2000). Contemporary Nutrition: Issues and Insights. U.S.A.: The McGraw-Hill Companies, Inc. (p.176-185)

15. https://www.verywellmind.com/what-is-serotonin-425327, By Kristalyn Salters

16. Pedneault, PhD
 Medically reviewed by Daniel B. Block, MD,

17. https://www.verywellmind.com/cortisol-and-stress-how-to-stay-healthy-3145080, By Elizabeth Scott, MS , Steven Gans, MD , Updated on February 21, 2020

18. https://www.webmd.com/healthy-aging/aging-dhea-test#1

19. https://www.google.com/search?q=Low+GABA&oq=Low+GAB-A&aqs=chrome.0.69i59j0l7.4402j0j4&sourceid=chrome&ie=UTF-861dsam

20. https://www.ncbi.nlm.nih.gov/pmc/articles/PMC4854098/

21. https://facty.com/ailments/body/10-symptoms-of-estrogen-dominance/?-style=quick&utm_source=adwords-ca&adid=409872377711&utm_medium=c-search&utm_term=estrogen%20dominance&utm_campaign=FHCA---Symptoms-of-High-Estro-gen---desktop&gclid=Cj0KCQjwmdzzBRC7ARIsANdqRRnYVDAWHRrtAEOhNQejXw-GtmMOL66kdwq5_ALXsa780eMtjb8BWqPgaAhNQEALw_wcB

22. Turner, Natasha. (2010). The Hormone Diet: Lose Fat, Gain Strength, Live Younger Longer. Toronto, Canada: Random House of Canada Limited.(pp.74-75)

23. https://www.mayoclinic.org/diseases-conditions/vaginal-atrophy/symptoms-causes/syc-20352288

24. https://www.healthline.com/health/womens-health/low-progesterone#low-progesterone

25. https://www.yourhormones.info/hormones/progesterone/

26. https://www.yourhormones.info/hormones/testosterone/ (Education Resource from the Society of Endocrinology)

27. https://www.performanceinsiders.com/sugar-affects-testosterone.html
28. https://craiglewisfitness.com/16-ways-to-increase-testosterone/

29. https://www.mdmag.com/medical-news/testosterone-replacement-therapy-linked-to-reducing-blood-sugar-levels

30. https://www.everlywell.com/discover/unhealthy-testosterone-levels-in-men

31. https://www.health.harvard.edu/diseases-and-conditions/the-lowdown-on-thyroid-slowdown, Harvard Health Publishing (Harvard Medical School)

32. Turner, Natasha. (2010). The Hormone Diet: Lose Fat, Gain Strength, Live Younger Longer. Toronto, Canada: Random House of Canada Limited. (pp.96-97)

33. https://www.atherosclerosis-journal.com/article/S0021-9150(19)30087-5/fulltext

34. https://www.google.com/search?q=Symptoms+of+high+cholesterol&oq=Symptoms+of+high+cholesterol&aqs=chrome..69i57j0l7.15749j0j9&sourceid=chrome&ie=UTF-8

35. Medically reviewed by Judith Marcin, MD on May 14, 2018 — Written by Rena Gold-manhttps://www.healthline.com/health/high-cholesterol/how-long-does-it-take-to-lower

36. ttps://www.google.com/search?q=too+much+fat+in+the+blood&oq=Too+much+fat+in+the+blood&aqs=chrome.0.0l8.108628j0j9&sourceid=chrome&ie=UTF-8

37. Written by Rachael Link, MS, RD on March 9, 2017, https://www.healthline.com/nutrition/13-ways-to-lower-triglycerides

38. Claire Delong; Sandeep Sharma. Physiology, Peripheral Vascular Resistance. February 7, 2019., ncbi.nlm.nih.gov/books/ NBK538308/

39. Tamilselvi Ramanathan, FRCA, Henry Skinner, FRCA. April 1, 2005. Coronary Blood Flow, Con-tinuing Education in Anaesthesia Critical Care & Pain, Volume 5, Issue 2, April 2005, Pages 61–64, https://doi.org/10.1093/bjaceaccp/mki012; https://academic.oup.com/bja-ed/article/5/2/61/422091

40. Amy Hess-Fischl MS, RD, LDN, BC-ADM, CDE, https://www.endocrineweb.com/conditions/type-1-diabetes/what-insulin

41. American Lung Association, https://www.lung.org/lung-health-diseases/how-lungs-work

Helping people rebuild from the inside out.

40. American Lung Association, https://www.lung.org/lung-health-diseases/how-lungs-work

41. Sharoon David; Sandeep Sharma, July 27, 2020. Vital Capacity, https://www.ncbi.nlm.nih.gov/books/NBK541099/

42. Pediatric Critical Care (Third Edition), 2006, https://www.sciencedirect.com/topics/medicine-and-dentistry/airway-resistance

43. https://kidshealth.org/en/parents/brain-nervous-system.html

44. Purves D, Augustine GJ, Fitzpatrick D, et al., editors, Sunderland (MA): Sinauer Associates; 2001.,
 Neuroscience. 2nd edition, https://www.ncbi.nlm.nih.gov/books/NBK11042/#:~:text=The%20brain%20receives%20blood%20from,anterior%20and%20middle%20cerebral%20arteries.

45. Medically reviewed by Elaine K. Luo, M.D. — Written by Shannon Johnson on October 10, 2019, https://www.medicalnewstoday.com/articles/326621#:~:text=The%20cranial%20nerves%20are%20a,see%2C%20smell%2C%20and%20hear.

46. Kendra Cherry, MD, Daniel B. Block, MD on May 15, 2020, What Is Memory, https://www.verywellmind.com/what-is-memory-2795006

47. American College of Rheumatology, https://www.rheumatology.org/I-Am-A/Patient-Caregiver/Diseases-Conditions/Rheumatoid-Arthritis#:~:text=Fast%20Facts,stop%20joint%20pain%20and%20swelling.

48. Steven R. Garfin, MD, Spinal Stenosis: Lumbar and Cervical, https://www.spineuniverse.com/conditions/spinal-stenosis/spinal-stenosis-lumbar-cervical#:~:text=As%20people%20age%2C%20the%20ligaments,occurs%20and%20leads%20to%20compression

49. Glenda Taylor, March 20, 2019, What are the LymphNodes

50. Louise Dunphy, Syed Hussain Abbas, Arjun Patel and Giovanni Tebala, Abstract, Spontaneous Splenic rupture: a rare first presentation of diffuse large B cell lymphoma, https://casereports.bmj.com/content/12/8/e231101?utm_source=google&utm_medium=cpc&utm_campaign=usage&utm_content=dynamic&utm_term=&gclid=Cj0KCQjw7ZL6BRCmARIsAH6XFDJUeioSbjk6UdZbFfcgdNb3xkisyvrgWKkO6emDqUQD-

v0OkQkJ-lboaAvSAEALw_wcB

51. Abhisek Dwivedy and Palok Aich, Abstract, Int J Gen Med. 2011; 4: 299–311. Published online 2011 Apr 12., doi: 10.2147/IJGM.S17525 , Importance of innate mucosal immunity and the promises it holds, https://www.ncbi.nlm.nih.gov/pmc/articles/PMC3085239/

52. Alkalosis, Medical Encyclopedia, MedlinePlus, https://medlineplus.gov/ency/article/001183.htm

53. Medically reviewed by Katherine Marengo LDN. R.D., Written by Zawn Villines, January 24, 2019, Medical News Today, https://www.medicalnewstoday.com/articles/324271

54. The Facts, Metal Hypersensitivity, https://medbroadcast.com/condition/getcondition/metal-hypersensitivity

55. Cedars-Sinai Staff Blog, Collagen for Your Skin: Healthy or Hype? https://www.cedars-sinai.org/blog/collagen-supplements.html#:~:text=Collagen%20is%20a%20protein%20that,-look%2C%22%20says%20dermatologist%20Dr.

56. Medically reviewed by Suzanne Falck, M.D., FACP — Written by Lana Barhum on May 21, 2018, What happens when calcium levels are low?, https://www.medicalnewstoday.com/articles/321865

57. Sandra M. McLachlan and Basil Rapoport, Endocr Rev. 2014 Feb; 35(1): 59–105. Published online 2013 Oct 3. doi: 10.1210/er.2013-1055, Breaking Tolerance to Thyroid Antigens: Changing Concepts in Thyroid Autoimmunity

58. National Library of Medicine, Lauric Acid, https://pubchem.ncbi.nlm.nih.gov/compound/Lauric-acid

59. Wikipedia, The Free Encyclopedia, Myristic Acid, https://en.wikipedia.org/wiki/Myristic_acid#:~:text=Myristic%20acid%20(IUPAC%20systematic%20name,to%20as%20myristates%20or%20tetradecanoates.

60. Palmitoleic Acid: A Complete Guide to This Omega-7 Fatty Acid, https://www.dropanfbomb.com/blogs/articles-resources/palmitoleic-acid

Helping people rebuild from the inside out.

61. https://www.google.com/search?q=Symptoms+of+high+cholesterol&oq=Symptoms+of+high+cholesterol&aqs=chrome..69i57j0l7.15749j0j9&sourceid=chrome&ie=UTF-8

62. https://www.google.com/search?q=too+much+fat+in+the+blood&oq=Too+much+-fat+in+the+blood&aqs=chrome.0.0l8.108628j0j9&sourceid=chrome&ie=UTF-8

63. Kyle S. McCommis, Thomas A. Goldstein, Dana R. Abendschein, Bernd Misselwitz, Thomas Pil-gram, Robert J. Gropler, and Jie Zheng, Published in final edited form as: Eur Radiol. 2010 Aug; 20(8): 2005–2012. Published online 2010 Feb 24., https://www.ncbi.nlm.nih.gov/pmc/articles/PMC2900455/

64. Lydia C. Boyette; Biagio Manna. Last Update: April 3, 2019., Physiology, Myocardial Oxygen Demand

65. National Institute of Diabetes and Digestive and Kidney Diseases, Symptoms & Causes of Dumping Syn-drome, https://www.niddk.nih.gov/health-information/digestive-diseases/dumping-syndrome/symptoms-causes

66. Motility Disorders, 02 October 2019, https://www.iffgd.org/gi-disorders/motility-disorders.html

67. Agata Matejuk, Abstract, Skin Immunity, Arch Immunol Ther Exp (Warsz). 2018; 66(1): 45–54.
Published online 2017 Jun 16. doi: 10.1007/s00005-017-0477-3, https://www.ncbi.nlm.nih.gov/pmc/articles/PMC5767194/

68. Author links open overlay panel Mary F.Bennett1Michael K.Robinson2Elma Daraon1Kevin D.Cooper1, Volume 13, Issue 1, April 2008, Pages 15-19, Journal of Investigative Dermatology Symposium Proceedings, https://www.sciencedirect.com/science/article/pii/S0022202X15526614,

69. Medically reviewed by Cynthia Cobb, DNP, APRN — Written by Corey Whelan, August 29, 2019, Skin Elasticity: 13 Ways to Improve It, https://www.healthline.com/health/beauty-skin-care/skin-elasticity

70. Robert D. Murray, in Williams Textbook of Endocrinology (Thirteenth Edition), 2016, The Long-Term Endocrine Sequelae of Multimodality Cancer Therapy, Gonadotropins, Science Direct, https://www.sciencedirect.com/topics/medicine-and-dentistry/gonadotropin-de-

ficiency

71. Cervicitis, Mayo Clinic, https://www.mayoclinic.org/diseases-conditions/cervicitis/symptoms-causes/syc-20370814

72. Medically reviewed by Debra Sullivan, Ph.D., MSN, R.N., CNE, COI — Written by Gretchen Holm - Up-dated on July 27, 2017, Underactive Pituitary Gland (Hypopituitarism), https://www.healthline.com/health/hypopituitarism

73. Topic Review, What is Tonsilitis, CIGNA, https://www.cigna.com/individuals-families/health-wellness/hw/medical-topics/tonsillitis-ut1026
74 Reticulocyte Count, https://medlineplus.gov/lab-tests/reticulocyte-count/

75. Medically reviewed by Cynthia Taylor Chavoustie, MPAS, PA-C — Written by Kathryn Watson — Updated on January 9, 2020, What is Lazy Bowel Syndrome?, Healthline, https://www.healthline.com/health/lazy-bowel

76. Dr. George Papanicolaou, DO, The Ultra Wellness Center, https://www.ultrawellness-center.com/2017/09/21/the-wrong-gut-bugs-can-make-you-fat-and-sick-and-how-to-fix-them/

www.ingramcontent.com/pod-product-compliance
Lightning Source LLC
Chambersburg PA
CBHW042353030426

42336CB00029B/3463